Vasculitis in Clinical Practice

Richard A. Watts
David G.I. Scott
Chetan Mukhtyar

Vasculitis in Clinical Practice

Second Edition

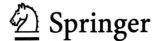 Springer

Richard A. Watts
Consultant Rheumatologist
and Honorary Senior Lecturer
Department of Rheumatology
Ipswich Hospital NHS Trust
Ipswich, UK

David G.I. Scott
Honorary Consultant
Rheumatologist and
Honorary Professor
Department of Rheumatology
Norfolk and Norwich
University Hospital
Norwich, UK

Chetan Mukhtyar
Consultant Rheumatologist
and Honorary Senior Lecturer
Department of Rheumatology
Norfolk and Norwich
University Hospital
Norwich, UK

ISBN 978-3-319-14870-0   ISBN 978-3-319-14871-7   (eBook)
DOI 10.1007/978-3-319-14871-7

Library of Congress Control Number: 2015940329

Springer Cham Heidelberg New York Dordrecht London
© Springer International Publishing AG, Cham 2015

Springer International Publishing AG Switzerland is part of Springer Science+Business Media (www.springer.com)

Preface

The systemic vasculitides are a group of disorders which are of increasing importance. Many of these conditions are only rarely encountered by general physicians and often present significant diagnostic challenges. Our goal in writing this short book was to provide easily accessible information in a pocket-sized format. We hope we have helped the general rheumatologist, who only encounters these problems occasionally. We have focused on clinical presentation, diagnostic processes, and current management. The second edition of the book has been updated to include current nomenclature and developments in treatment since the publication of the first edition. We hope, therefore, that we will help our patients with these potentially devastating conditions by improving diagnosis and therapy.

Ipswich, UK   Richard A. Watts
Norwich, UK   David G.I. Scott
Norwich, UK   Chetan Mukhtyar

Contents

Chapter Overview

Part I
Introduction

Chapter 1
Definitions

1.1 General Introduction

The systemic vasculitides are relatively uncommon but important conditions which cause significant morbidity and mortality and often confusion at first presentation to a broad spectrum of clinicians. Recent advances in treatment have made it possible for most conditions to be effectively controlled and sometimes even cured. Thirty or forty years ago, these were diseases with a high mortality, but the introduction of appropriate immunosuppressive treatment has changed the outcome for most patients, such that they are now part of the spectrum of chronic inflammatory diseases requiring ongoing treatment and monitoring.

The aim of this book is to provide easy access to the common clinical presentations of the systemic vasculitides, the investigations required to assess the severity of the disease as well as diagnose specific vasculitic syndromes and an approach to treatment based on the important studies undertaken over the last 15 years, particularly within Europe, using conventional immunosuppressive drugs and also more recent studies looking at the role of modern biologic therapy.

There have been major changes in our understanding of the effects of treatment of vasculitis. Recently completed studies described in this book, involve the current use of intravenous pulse cyclophosphamide which is almost as

R.A. Watts et al., *Vasculitis in Clinical Practice*,
DOI 10.1007/978-3-319-14871-7_1,
© Springer International Publishing AG, Cham 2015

effective as continuous oral cyclophosphamide but safer and the role of B-cell depletion which is as effective in inducing remission as cyclophosphamide, but with potentially less long term toxicity. Azathioprine and methotrexate are equally effective in maintaining remission after induction remission with cyclophosphamide and/or B cell depletion. At present there is also convincing evidence that patients with particularly severe systemic vasculitis (especially those with severe renal and pulmonary disease) are more responsive to plasma exchange as compared to intravenous methylprednisolone.

The long-term outcome for most vasculitides has substantially improved over the last two or three decades but there is still an early mortality (as high as 5 or 10 %) in the case of anti-neutrophil cytoplasmic antibody (ANCA) associated vasculitis. As outlined above, vasculitis is usually brought under control with intensive immunosuppression and maintained by lower dose/less intensive drug treatment and then it is seen as a more chronic, sometimes relapsing disease with an accumulative mortality and morbidity which after 10 years or so may be influenced by an increased cardiovascular risk.

In conclusion, the systemic vasculitides are an important group of diseases. Patients with systemic vasculitis exhaust significant health service resources because of the severity of the disease at onset. They are potentially treatable and controllable diseases so early recognition and early treatment, particularly before significant renal damage has occurred, is important. Later relapses involving the kidney will inevitably lead to renal failure if the disease is left uncontrolled, and so these are diseases that not only need careful monitoring and treatment in the longer term but also aggressive immunosuppression at presentation.

1.2   Definitions

Recent changes have been made to the nomenclature of some of the vasculitides; these include Granulomatosis with Polyangiitis (GPA formerly known as Wegener's granulomatosis), Eosinophilic Granulomatosis with Polyangiitis (EGPA formerly called Churg–Strauss syndrome) and IgA Vasculitis (formerly known as Henoch–Schönlein purpura).

They all form part of a heterogeneous group of conditions that can occur independently (for example GPA (Wegeners), and microscopic polyangiitis (MPA)) or as a complication of an established disease such as rheumatoid arthritis, or systemic lupus erythematosus. The word "vasculitis" means that the "itis" or inflammation is directed at the blood vessel wall, and the consequence of such inflammation is damage and destruction to the vessel wall seen histologically as fibrinoid necrosis; hence the term "necrotizing vasculitis" has often been used in the past. Vasculitis may be localized to a single organ or vascular bed, where it is relatively benign but, more commonly, generalized. Small muscular arteries can develop focal or segmental lesions which may be life-threatening. The event of the former affecting part of the vessel wall can lead to aneurysm formation and possible rupture whereas segmental lesions affect the whole circumference and are more common but lead to stenosis or occlusion with distal infarction. The consequence of vasculitis depends on the site, size and number of blood vessels involved. These pathological processes explain why severe hemorrhage and vital organ infarction are the major consequences and life-threatening complications of systemic vasculitis. When only very small vessels (capillaries, venules) are involved, as occurs in some small vessel vasculitides, the organ most commonly affected is the skin and this causes problems only when sufficient numbers of blood vessels are involved, compromising tissue perfusion, or when there is severe inflammatory response associated with it (especially where the kidney is involved).

The terminology used for vasculitis is confusing. The term necrotizing vasculitis as outlined above reflects histology, as does leucocytoclastic vasculitis, which indicates a pathological process where there is extravasation of red blood cells and neutrophil debris within the inflammatory infiltrate around the blood vessel. Leucocytoclasis is most commonly seen in pure small vessel vasculitis but can be a feature of larger vessel disease; for example, leucocytoclasis is not uncommon in the arterial wall of patients with polyarteritis nodosa.

Other terms that are currently used include primary systemic vasculitis and ANCA-associated vasculitis. The term primary vasculitis differentiates vasculitis occurring de novo as outlined above, with vasculitis occurring as a secondary event, either to a known cause such as viral infection (hepatitis B, C, etc.), connective tissue disease such as rheumatoid arthritis or systemic lupus erythematosus, and also associated with some types of malignancy. Primary systemic vasculitis is also a term often used to describe medium and small vessel disease and usually excludes, for example, small vessel vasculitis such as IgA Vasculitis or the larger vessel arteritides such as Kawasaki disease and giant cell arteritis.

After the description of ANCA in the mid 1980s, there has been an explosion in our understanding of the autoimmune process involved in vasculitis, and these diseases are now considered to be part of the autoimmune spectrum. The clinical syndromes most strongly associated with ANCA are GPA (Wegener's) (associated with ANCA with PR3 specificity) and MPA (microscopic polyangiitis, associated with ANCA with myeloperoxidase (MPO) specificity). Sometimes included in this group is EGPA (Churg–Strauss syndrome) in which about 40–50 % of patients have ANCA, usually MPO, especially in those with renal involvement.. ANCA may also be seen in patients with renal limited vasculitis – that is with patients whose disease appears to involve the kidney only and without some of the other systemic features. These patients are more like those with MPA, but they must also be included when the term ANCA-associated vasculitis is used.

Chapter 2
Classification
and Epidemiology

2.1 Introduction

The classification of vasculitis has been an area of controversy for many years, with specific classification criteria only introduced relatively recently. Kussmaul and Maier [1] provided the first description of "periarteritis nodosa" when they described a patient with a systemic illness characterized by numerous nodules along the course of small muscular arteries.

The most widely accepted classification system reflects dominant vessel size and association with antineutrophil cytoplasmic antibodies (ANCA) (Table 2.1). This classification system also broadly reflects the therapeutic approaches that are applied to the different groups. The medium and small vessel group respond well to immunosuppression with cyclophosphamide and corticosteroids, whereas the large vessel group require moderate to high dose steroids and the small vessel group only sometimes require low dose corticosteroids. Also, the small-medium vessel group is the most likely to develop glomerulonephritis and renal failure, is associated with ANCA, and contrast pathogenetically with the small vessel group, which is often associated with immune complexes. This has led to the emergence of the concept of ANCA-associated vasculitis (AAV) which reflects the notion that granulomatosis with polyangiitis (Wegener's) (GPA), microscopic polyangiitis

R.A. Watts et al., *Vasculitis in Clinical Practice*,
DOI 10.1007/978-3-319-14871-7_2,
© Springer International Publishing AG, Cham 2015

TABLE 2.1 Classification of systemic vasculitis

Dominant vessel involved	Primary	Secondary
Large arteries	Giant cell arteritis (GCA) Takayasu arteritis (TAK)	Aortitis associated with RA Infection (e.g., syphilis, tuberculosis)
Medium arteries	Kawasaki disease Polyarteritis nodosa (PAN)	Hepatitis B virus associated PAN
Small ANCA associated	Granulomatosis with polyangiitis (Wegener's) (GPA) Eosinophilic granulomatosis with polyangiitis (Churg–Strauss) (EGPA) Microscopic polyangiitis (MPA)	Drugs[a]
Small Immune complex	IgA Vasculitis (Henoch–Schönlein purpura) (IgAV) Cryoglobulinaemic vasculitis (non-HCV) Anti-GBM disease Hypocomplementaemic vasculitis	RA, SLE, Sjogren's syndrome Serum sickness Cryoglobulinaemic vasculitis (HCV associated) Drug induced[b]
Variable	Behçet's Cogan's syndrome	Drugs[c]

RA rheumatoid arthritis, *PAN* polyarteritis nodosa, *SLE* systemic lupus erythematosus

[a]Most commonly propylthiouracil, hydralazine which may induce an ANCA-associated vasculitis (AAV) typically MPO-ANCA
[b]For example, sulfonamides, penicillins, thiazide diuretics and many others
[c]For example, cocaine

(MPA) and eosinophilic granulomatosis with polyangiitis (Churg–Strauss) (EGPA) share many features in common and they are often included together in clinical trials.

2.2   ACR (1990) Criteria

The American College of Rheumatology (ACR), in 1990, proposed the criteria for the classification of seven different vasculitides (Giant cell arteritis (GCA), Takayasu arteritis (TAK),
GPA, EGPA, Polyarteritis Nodosa (PAN), IgA vasculitis
(Henoch–Schönlein) (IgAV), Hypersensitivity vasculitis (HSV))
with sensitivities varying from 71.0 to 95.3 % and specificities of
78.7–99.7 % [2]. The most sensitive and specific criteria were
found in EGPA, GCA, and TAK; hypersensitivity (leukocytoclastic) vasculitis was the least well-defined condition. The ACR
criteria have a number of drawbacks. The criteria were developed before the wide spread introduction of ANCA. They do
not include MPA, which was a term not in common use during
the 1980s. It is important to stress that they were designed as
classification criteria and not diagnostic criteria.

2.3   Chapel Hill Consensus Definitions

In 1994, the Chapel Hill Consensus conference (CHCC)
introduced definitions for vasculitis [3]. They included MPA,
but were not intended either as classification or diagnostic
criteria. They recognized that histological data would not be
available for all patients especially when the clinical condition of the patient might preclude obtaining appropriate
biopsies or the sample might not be representative and
miss salient histological features. The concept of surrogate
markers of vasculitis was therefore introduced, but a list
of markers was not provided. In addition, the importance of
ANCA in diagnosis was recognized. However neither surrogate markers nor ANCA were included in the definitions.

The CHCC 1994 definitions were updated in 2012 [4]. The
modifications included an expanded list of defined conditions, the recognition that the ANCA associated vasculitides
formed a separate group and introduced new names for some
conditions to recognize increased knowledge of aetiopatho-
genesis. Table 2.1 incorporates the new hierarchy.

2.4   EMEA Algorithm

The lack of consistency between the ACR criteria and the CHCC (1994) definitions led to the development of a consensus algorithm in an attempt to provide a consistent approach for the purposes of epidemiological studies. (Fig. 2.1) [5] The algorithm uses a hierarchical approach starting with EGPA. EGPA was considered first because the ACR criteria have a high specificity and sensitivity. Next GPA was considered, then MPA and finally PAN. The aim was to have a minimum of unclassifiable patients. Although ANCA was included the specificity was not associated with type of vasculitis. The algorithm was validated and has been shown to be unaffected by the changes introduced by the CHCC in 2012 [6].

2.5   Epidemiology

The systemic vasculitides are generally diseases of childhood or old age (Fig. 2.2) [7]. Kawasaki disease occurs almost exclusively in children aged <2 years and very rarely over the age of 5 years (900/million/year children aged <5 years). IgAV has a peak age of incidence in adolescence, but occurs less frequently in adults. At the other end of the age spectrum, the AAV occur with a peak age of onset in those aged 65–75 years, while GCA has a peak age of onset in those aged over 80 years. Other types of vasculitis are much rarer; TAK occurs in those aged less than 40 years.

The epidemiology of vasculitis has been mainly studied in Caucasian white populations, there being relatively little data from other ethnic groups. GCA appears to be most common in populations of Scandinavian descent and relatively uncommon in Africans and Japanese. TAK by contrast is generally believed to be more common in Japan than Europe. The AAV show a relatively uniform overall incidence (20/million/year) in the populations studied but the distribution of GPA, MPA and EGPA differs. In Europe, for instance in the North, GPA is more common than MPA, whereas in Southern

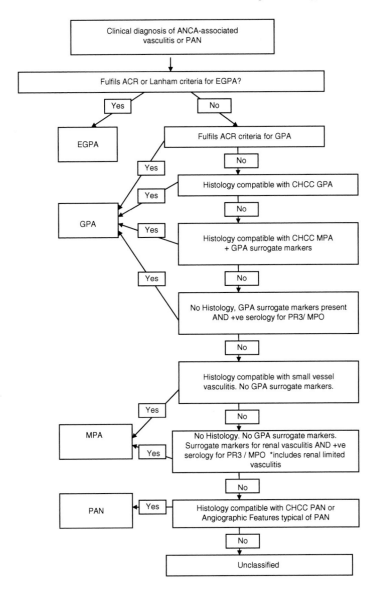

FIGURE 2.1 EMEA Algorithm for classification of vasculitis (Reproduced with permission from BMJ Publishing Group Ltd)

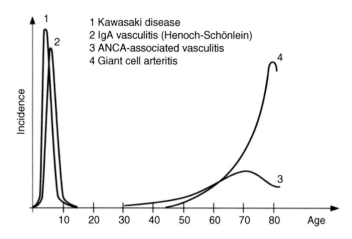

FIGURE 2.2 Relative incidence of vasculitis by age (By permission of Oxford University Press)

Europe the reverse occurs. MPA is more common than GPA in South East Asian populations. In the UK, KD is more common in Asians of Indian descent than Afro-caribbeans and white Caucasians. Similarly IgAV is more common in Asians than White Caucasians.

2.6   Etiological Factors

In general the cause of vasculitis is unknown. The key event being the interaction of an environmental agent (unknown) with a genetically predisposed host. At present relatively little is known about the genetic factors which are important. HLA type is an important risk factor for several types of vasculitis e.g. HLA DR1*0401 and GPA, HLA B51 and Behçet's disease. Infection has long been considered an important trigger but except for a few specific instances no causal relationship has been established (e.g., HBV and PAN, HCV, and cryoglobulinemia). Numerous drugs have been implicated, but hydralazine and propylthiouracil are clearly implicated in the development of MPO-ANCA vasculitis.

Key Points
- Diagnostic classification of vasculitis is difficult as there are no validated criteria.
- The vasculitides are conditions of extremes of age.
- Giant cell arteritis (GCA) is the most common systemic vasculitis.

References

1. Kussmaul A, Maier R. Über eine bisher nicht beschriebene eigentümliche Arterienerkrankung (Periarteritis nodosa), die mit Morbus Brightü und rapid fortschreitender allgemeiner Muskellähmung einhergeht. Deutsche Archive Klinical Medizine. 1866;1:484–514.
2. Fries JF, Hunder GG, Bloch DA, et al. The American College of Rheumatology 1990 criteria for the classification of vasculitis. Summary. Arthritis Rheum. 1990;33:1135–6.
3. Jennette JC, Falk RJ, Andrassy K, et al. Nomenclature of systemic vasculitides. Proposal of an international consensus conference. Arthritis Rheum. 1994;37:187–92.
4. Jennette JC, Falk RJ, Bacon PA, et al. 2012 Revised international Chapel Hill Consensus Conference nomenclature of vasculitides. Arthritis Rheum. 2013;65:1–11.
5. Watts R, Lane S, Hanslik T, Hauser T, Hellmich B, Koldingsnes W, et al. Development and validation of a consensus methodology for the classification of the ANCA-associated vasculitides and polyarteritis nodosa for epidemiological studies. Ann Rheum Dis. 2007;66(2):222–7.
6. Abdulkader R, Lane SE, Scott DGI, Watts RA. Classification of vasculitis: EMA classification using CHCC 2012 definitions. Ann Rheum Dis. 2013;72(11):1888.
7. Watts RA, Scott DGI. Epidemiology of vasculitis. In: Ball GV, Fessler BJ, Bridges SL, editors. Oxford textbook of vasculitis. 3rd ed. Oxford: Oxford University Press; 2014. p. 7–25.

Chapter 3
General Presentation of the Vasculitides

3.1 Introduction

Primary systemic vasculitis can involve the vasculature of any organ-system. Depending on the calibre of the vessels involved and the organs affected, vasculitis can present in a myriad of ways to a number of specialties. There are no diagnostic criteria or pathognomonic laboratory investigations for systemic vasculitis. The application of classification criteria in clinical practice have been disappointing and should be avoided. The classification criteria of the American College of Rheumatology had a positive predictive value of 17–29 % in a cohort of patients with a differential diagnosis of systemic vasculitis [1]. The Chapel Hill nomenclature is similarly unsatisfactory [2]. Histopathology can be diagnostic, but has variable diagnostic yield depending on the skill of the operator, method of sampling, and the organ biopsied [3, 4].

3.2 Pattern Recognition

In the absence of assistance from laboratory tests or diagnostic criteria, recognition of clinical patterns supported by laboratory tests is of value in the diagnosis of systemic vasculitis. Table 3.1 provides examples of presentation patterns of specific vasculitic syndromes [5]. The table illustrates the value of

R.A. Watts et al., *Vasculitis in Clinical Practice*,
DOI 10.1007/978-3-319-14871-7_3,
© Springer International Publishing AG, Cham 2015

TABLE 3.1 Common clinical patterns of vasculitis

Examples of presentation	Possible diagnosis
Recurrent sinonasal disease with or without septal perforation, orbital involvement (radiological or clinical)	Granulomatosis with polyangiitis
A pulmonary syndrome on the background of chronic poorly controlled asthma with peripheral eosinophilia with or without a peripheral neuropathy	Eosinophilic granulomatosis with polyangiitis
Pulmonary-renal syndrome: microscopic haematuria, hypertension, renal impairment, dyspnoea, haemoptysis	Granulomatosis with polyangiitis or microscopic polyangiitis
Vasculitic rash, ulcer, neuropathy on the background of hepatitis or the presence of liver abnormalities at presentation	Cryoglobulinaemic vasculitis
Purpuric lesions mainly on the extensor surface of the lower limbs including gluteal involvement with or without microscopic hematuria, arthritis and abdominal pain	IgA vasculitis
Multiple constitutional symptoms, leg ulcers, orchitis, abdominal pain, hypertension without evidence of glomerular or alveolar involvement	Polyarteritis nodosa
A new onset headache in individuals above the age of 50 with temporal artery or scalp tenderness and raised ESR	Giant cell arteritis
New-onset vascular claudication in any limb with peripheral pulse abnormalities in an individual less than 40 years of age	Takayasu's arteritis

TABLE 3.1 (continued)

Examples of presentation	Possible diagnosis
Acute onset of fever, desquamating rash and mucocutaneous lymphadenopathy in a toddler	Kawasaki's disease
Orogenital ulceration, hypopyon, uveitis, arthritis in a young male of Mediterranean descent	Behçet's disease
Constitutional symptoms, raised inflammatory markers, patchy aortic and/or periaortic inflammation with hepato-biliary or pancreatic involvement	IgG4 related disease

Adapted from Nataraja et al. [5]

a structured clinical interview and examination at presentation and follow-up. The rarity of systemic vasculitis and the multisystem nature of the pathology often cause delay in diagnosis. The Birmingham Vasculitis Activity Score is a validated clinical tool to quantify disease activity in patients with systemic vasculitis [6]. It is a single A4 sheet listing common or important manifestations of systemic vasculitis. The author uses it to quantify disease activity in clinical practice, but it also serves as an aide memoire of clinical manifestations to check for patients with a suspicion of systemic vasculitis (Table 3.2).

It is important to perform a thorough clinical examination at each interview in patients with established disease, as new clinical manifestations may emerge late in the disease.

3.3   Laboratory Investigations

In patients with clinical suspicion of systemic vasculitis, the following laboratory investigations provide useful diagnostic information.

TABLE 3.2 The Birmingham Vasculitis Activity Score showing a list of clinically important and relevant manifestations of systemic vasculitis

Birmingham Vasculitis Activity Score (version 3)

Patient ID:	Date of birth:	Total score:
Assessor:	Date of assessment:	

Tick an item only if attributable to active vasculitis. If there are no abnormalities in a section, please tick 'None' for that organ-system.	If all abnormalities are due to persistent disease (active vasculitis which is not new/worse in the prior 4 weeks), tick the **PERSISTENT** box at the bottom right corner

Is this the patient's first assessment? Yes ○				No ○	
	None	Active disease		None	Active disease
1. General	○		**6. Cardiovascular**	○	
Myalgia		○	Lossof pulses		○
Arthralgia/arthritis		○	Valvular heart disease		○
Fever ≥38°C		○	Pericarditis		○
Weight loss >? kg		○	Ischaemic cardiac pain		○
			Cardiomyopathy		○
2. Cutaneous	○		Congestive cardiac failure		○
Infarct		○			
Purpura		○	**7. Abdominal**	○	
Ulcer		○	Peritonitis		○
Gangrene		○	Bloody diarrhoea		○
Other skin vasculitis		○	Ischaemic abdominal pain		○
3. Mucous membranes / eyes	○		**8. Renal**	○	
Mouth ulcers		○	Hypertension		○
Genital ulcers		○	Proteinuria >1+		○
Adnexal inflammation		○	Haematuria ≥10 RBCs/hpf		○
Significant proptosis		○	Serum creatinine 125-249 μmol/L*		○
Scleritis / Episcleritis		○	Serum creatinine 250-499 μmol/L*		○
Conjunctivitis / Episcleritis / Keratitis		○	Serum creatinine ≥500 μmol/L*		○
Blurred vision		○	Rise in serum creatinine >30% or fall in creatinine clearence > 25%		○
Sudden visual loss		○	*Can only be scored on the first assessment		
Uveitis		○			
Retinal changes (vasculitis / thrombosis / exuclate / haemorrhage)		○			

TABLE 3.2 (continued)

4. Renal	○		9. Nervous system	○	
Bloody nasal discharge / crusts / ulcers / granulomata		○	Headache		○
			Meningitis		○
Paranasal sinus Involvement		○	Organic confusion		○
			Seizures (not hypertensive)		○
Subglottic stenosis		○	Cerebrovascular accident		○
Conductive hearing loss		○	Spinal cord lesion		○
Sensorineural hearing loss		○	Cranial nerve palsy		○
			Sensory peripheral neuropathy		○
			Mononeuritis multiplex		○
5. Chest	○		10. Other	○	
Wheeze		○	a.		○
Nodules or cavities		○	b.		○
Pleural effusion / pleurisy		○	c.		○
			d.		○
Infiltrate		○			
Endobronchial involvement		○			
Massive haemoptysis / alveolar haemorrhage		○	**PERSISTENT DISEASE ONLY:**	☐	
Respiratory failure		○	(Tick here if all the abnormalities are due to persistent disease)		

Version 1: Luqmani et al. [8]
Version 2: Luqmani et al. [9]
Version 3: Mukhtyar et al. [6]. Reproduced with permission from BMJ Publishing Group Ltd

1. *Complete blood count* – Leukocytosis, neutrophilia, and a high platelet count are all acute phase reactants. Eosinophilia is seen in over 80 % of patients with Churg–Strauss syndrome. Leukopenia is uncommon and generally due to treatment.
2. *Renal function* – Serum creatinine may be abnormal in patients with small vessel disease due to inflammation of the afferent and efferent arterioles. In medium and large vessel disease, renal arterial or suprarenal aortic involvement may compromise renal function. Urine analysis demonstrating red cell casts is a sign of glomerular disease, and analysis should be performed immediately on the suspicion of systemic vasculitis. Urinary protein estimation

should be done early in the management of systemic vasculitis using urine protein/creatinine ratio.

3. *Liver function* – Viral hepatitis due to HBV and HCV is associated with polyarteritis nodosa and cryoglobulinemic vasculitis. Liver transaminases and alkaline phosphatase are often abnormal.

4. *Inflammatory markers* – The erythrocyte sedimentation rate and the C-reactive protein are usually elevated in systemic vasculitis. Normal levels should prompt an alternative explanation of the clinical manifestations.

5. *Immunology tests*

    (a) Antineutrophil cytoplasmic antibody directed against proteinase 3 and myeloperoxidase have a high specificity and sensitivity for the diagnosis of small vessel vasculitis in the appropriate clinical context [7] (Figs. 3.1 and 3.2).

    (b) Rheumatoid factor in high titers may be present in cryoglobulinemic vasculitis.

    (c) Complement (C3 and C4) consumption can suggest cryoglobulinemic vasculitis and hypocomplementemic urticarial vasculitis. Secondary vasculitis due to connective tissue diseases also demonstrates low C3 and C4 levels.

    (d) Immunoglobulin subclass testing may demonstrate raised IgG4 levels. These strongly suggest IgG4 related disease, but have been elevated in patients with ANCA associated vasculitis.

6. *Histopathology* – Biopsy can be diagnostic of systemic vasculitis but the yield can depend on the organ sampled and the skill of the operator. Example – kidney biopsies are positive in over 80 % of patients with renal involvement in ANCA-associated vasculitis [3], but otolaryngological biopsy has a low yield [4].

7. *Imaging* – Imaging plays an important role in the demonstration of solid-organ involvement, intramural and luminal vascular involvement, and infiltrative involvement from a granulomatous process. This will be dealt in greater detail in the individual sections.

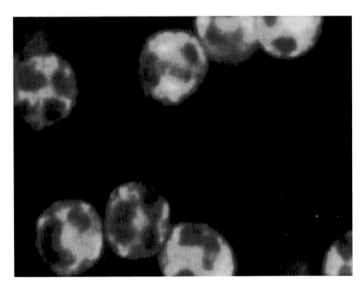

FIGURE 3.1 Indirect immunofluorescence of human neutrophils showing the typical cytoplasmic staining pattern of cANCA

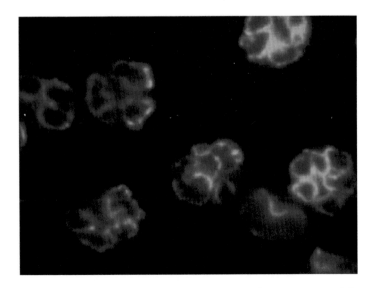

FIGURE 3.2 Indirect immunofluorescence of human neutrophils showing the typical perinuclear staining pattern of pANCA

3.4   Differential Diagnosis

The differential diagnosis of systemic vasculitis is broad. Infection and malignancy should always be ruled out. Chapters 15 and 16 deal with this in greater detail.

Key Points
- Vasculitis can present with protean manifestations involving many different organs.
- Vasculitis should be considered in differential diagnosis of any patient presenting with multisystem disease.
- Immunology markers are helpful in making the diagnosis when used in the appropriate clinical context.

References

1. Rao JK, Allen NB, Pincus T. Limitations of the 1990 American College of Rheumatology classification criteria in the diagnosis of vasculitis. Ann Intern Med. 1998;129:345–52.
2. Watts RA, Jolliffe VA, Carruthers DM, Lockwood CM, Scott DG. Effect of classification on the incidence of polyarteritis nodosa and microscopic polyangiitis. Arthritis Rheum. 1996;39:1208–12.
3. Aasarod K, Bostad L, Hammerstrom J, Jorstad S, Iversen BM. Renal histopathology and clinical course in 94 patients with Wegener's granulomatosis. Nephrol Dial Transplant. 2001;16:953–60.
4. Maguchi S, Fukuda S, Takizawa M. Histological findings in biopsies from patients with cytoplasmic-antineutrophil cytoplasmic antibody (cANCA)-positive Wegener's granulomatosis. Auris Nasus Larynx. 2001;28 Suppl 1:S53–8.
5. Nataraja A, Mukhtyar C, Hellmich B, Langford C, Luqmani R. Outpatient assessment of systemic vasculitis. Best Pract Res Clin Rheumatol. 2007;21:713–32.
6. Mukhtyar C, Lee R, Brown D, et al. Modification and validation of the Birmingham vasculitis activity score (Version 3). Ann Rheum Dis. 2009;68(12):1827–32.

7. Choi HK, Liu S, Merkel PA, Colditz GA, Niles JL. Diagnostic performance of antineutrophil cytoplasmic antibody tests for idiopathic vasculitides: metaanalysis with a focus on antimyeloperoxidase antibodies. J Rheumatol. 2001;28:1584–90.

8. Luqmani RA, et al. Birmingham Vasculitis Activity Score (BVAS) in systemic necrotizing. QJM. 1994;87(11):671–8.

9. Luqmani RA, et al. Disease assessment and management of the vasculitides. Baillieres Clin Rheumatol. 1997;11(2):423–46.

Chapter 4
General Principles of Treatment

4.1 Treatment

The type of vasculitis and the extent of organ involvement guide treatment. The intensity of initial immunosuppression depends on the severity of organ involvement and the size of the vessels involved (Table 4.1). Therefore, an important part of treatment planning involves the assessment of organ involvement and its severity. Treatment may be divided into remission induction, maintenance, and long-term follow-up. Guidelines on the management of the vasculitides have been recently published [1–3]. In this chapter, we will cover the general principles of treatment and the agents used.

4.2 Remission Induction

Remission induction covers the period of treatment from the initiation of therapy to remission. The choice of remission induction treatment depends on the severity of organ involvement and the size of the vessels involved (Table 4.1).

4.2.1 Large Vessel Disease

In general, large vessel vasculitis can be treated with oral prednisolone. Both TAK and GCA should be treated with

R.A. Watts et al., *Vasculitis in Clinical Practice*,
DOI 10.1007/978-3-319-14871-7_4,
© Springer International Publishing AG, Cham 2015

TABLE 4.1 Relationship between vessel size and response to induction treatment

Dominant vessel	Glucocorticoids alone	Cyclophosphamide/ glucocorticoids	Rituximab	Other treatments
Large arteries	+++	−	−	+
Medium arteries	+	++	−	++
Small vessels (ANCA)	+	+++	+++	+
Small vessels (IC)	+	+/−	+	++

high-dose oral glucocorticoids such as oral prednisolone (0.5–1.0 mg/kg). Sight threatening GCA may be treated with IV methyl prednisolone (1 g) [2]. Low-dose aspirin should be used in all patients with GCA unless contraindicated.

4.2.2 Medium Vessel Disease

Medium vessel vasculitis will require immunosuppressive therapy. Polyarteritis nodosa if associated with HBV infection should be treated as an infectious disease with plasma exchange and antiviral agents. Non-HBV-associated PAN will require immunosuppression with glucocorticoids and cyclophosphamide following the same approach for AAV [3].

Kawasaki disease is treated using intravenous immunoglobulin usually combined with glucocorticoids.

4.2.3 Medium/Small Vessel Vasculitis

The ANCA vasculitides are the major form of medium/small vessel vasculitis. Treatment is based on the severity of disease and the extent of organ involvement.

An algorithm has been developed to guide treatment for the medium/small ANCA-associated vasculitis (Fig. 4.1).

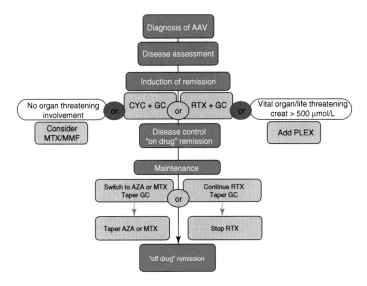

FIGURE 4.1 Algorithm for the introduction of treatment of ANCA-associated vasculitis (From Ntatsaki et al. [1], by permission of Oxford University Press)

Cyclophosphamide (CYC) is usually given intravenously (see Sect. 4.7.1) [1–3]. Rituximab may be used as an alternative induction agent to CYC.

4.2.4   Small Vessel Vasculitis

Many patients with isolated small vessel vasculitis especially when confined to the skin do not require treatment with glucocorticoids as the condition will be self limiting. A minority of children with IgAV (e.g., with renal involvement) will require immunosuppression with glucocorticoids (see Chap. 12).

4.3   Maintenance Therapy

Long-term maintenance therapy is mainly required for patients with AAV. Current clinical practice considers possible transfer to maintenance therapy as early as 3 months and aims for a maximum duration of CYC therapy of 6–12 months when successful remission has been achieved [4].

In patients with AAV who have achieved successful remission (usually between 3 and 6 months), cyclophosphamide should be withdrawn and substituted with either azathioprine in combination with oral steroids [4, 5]. Methotrexate, mycophenolate or leflunomide may be used as alternatives for intolerance or lack of efficacy of AZA. Azathioprine is the conventional choice for remission maintenance. Methotrexate, mycophenolate and leflunomide have not been shown to be superior to azathioprine and should be considered in azathioprine-intolerant patients. The role and optimum regimen for rituximab during maintenance is currently being evaluated, initial data suggests a role for 6 monthly infusion over a 2 year period (Mainritsan). During maintenance, glucocorticoids are tapered to prednisolone 15 mg/day (maximum) at 3 months, 10 mg/day (maximum) at 6 months, and 5 mg/day (maximum) at 12–18 months.

4.4   Long-Term Follow-Up

For many types of vasculitis, long-term follow is necessary, because there is a permanent risk of relapse even many years after diagnosis and successful remission induction. Drug toxicity, especially bladder carcinoma, may become apparent only many years after the completion of cyclophosphamide therapy, and regular urine dip stick must be performed.

4.5   Relapsing Disease

Relapses are classified as minor or major, according to the absence or presence of threatened vital organ function. Minor relapse is treated with an increase in prednisolone dose up to 30 mg/day, then gradual tapering and optimization of the concurrent immunosuppressive dose. Major relapse is treated with rituximab or cyclophosphamide using a similar regimen to primary remission induction, and an increase in prednisolone up to 0.5–1.0 mg/kg, maximum 1 g, intravenous methyl prednisolone or plasma exchange may be considered. Rituximab is used in preference to cyclophosphamide where the cumulative cyclophosphamide dose exceeds 15 g. In AAV, GPA is more likely to relapse than MPA. Persistence of positive ANCA is associated with an increased risk of relapse if treatment is withdrawn.

4.6 Refractory Disease

Disease refractory to induction with full-dose cyclophosphamide and prednisolone is rare. More commonly, optimal doses are not tolerated, or a prolonged relapsing disease course with high cumulative exposure to cyclophosphamide and prednisolone are the indications for alternative agents. Rituximab should be used in patients refractory to CYC. Other agents that could be considered include deoxyspergualin, and abatacept.

Intravenous immunoglobulin (IVIg) may be considered as an alternative therapy in patients with refractory disease or in patients for whom conventional therapy is contraindicated, e.g., in the presence of infection, in the severely ill patient, or in pregnancy. IVIg is effective, but only as a temporary measure and published data suggests that this lasts for about 3 months. T-cell depletion with antithymocyte globulin and pan-lymphocyte depletion with CAMPATH 1H (alemtuzumab, anti-CD52) have led to sustained remissions in refractory disease. TNF blockade has not been shown to be as effective as adjunctive therapy in clinical trials of AAV, but may have some steroid-sparing effect.

In the management of refractory vasculitis, it is important to identify the drivers for vasculitis, such as, intercurrent infection or malignancy, or noncompliance.

4.7 Specific Drugs Used to Treat Vasculitis

4.7.1 Cyclophosphamide

Cyclophosphamide is the induction agent of choice for the treatment of most patients with organ threatening disease

TABLE 4.2 Pulsed cyclophosphamide reductions for renal function and age

Age (years)	Creatinine 150–300 µmol/L	Creatinine 300–500 µmol/L
<60	15 mg/kg/pulse	12.5 mg/kg/pulse
>60 and <70	12.5 mg/kg/pulse	10 mg/kg/pulse
>70	10 mg/kg/pulse	7.5 mg/kg/pulse

(see Fig. 4.1) and should be combined with glucocorticoids. Cyclophosphamide is given using a pulse intravenous regimen [6]. Initially, pulses (15 mg/kg, maximum 1,000 mg) are given at 2 weekly and then 3 weekly intervals. Dose reductions should be made for age and renal function (Table 4.2) [6]. CYC may also be given as continuous low-dose oral treatment 2 mg/kg/day, maximum 200 mg/day. There is no difference in remission rates and no increased risk of relapse between the IV and oral regimens [6]. Continuous low dose oral CYC is associated with higher total CYC dosage and a significant higher infection risk. The cumulative dose of CYC was lower for the IV pulse regimen than for the continuous oral regimen when administered for the same period of time.

4.7.2   Glucocorticoids

Glucocorticoids are usually given as daily oral prednisolone. Glucocorticoids in combination with standard immune suppression are useful for the early control of disease activity in AAV, but are ineffective as sole therapy. The recommended regimen is based on that used in the published randomized trial of maintenance therapy for vasculitis [4]. The initial dose is 0.5–1 mg/kg up to 60 mg with rapid tapering down to 10 mg over a 6-month period and then more gradual tapering over the next 12–18 months. In patients with life-threatening disease or organ involvement, IV methylprednisolone (250–1,000 mg) may be used at the start of treatment and then oral prednisolone is continued.

4.7.3   Rituximab

Rituximab is a monoclonal anti-CD20 antibody which depletes B cells. Two recent RCTs have demonstrated that rituximab is not inferior to CYC in remission induction [7, 8]. It was more effective at remission induction in relapsing patients. Rituximab is the preferred agent for relapsing patients who have had more than 15 g cyclophosphamide, those at high risk of infection, and high risk of infertility. The clinical trials were conducted using 375 mg/m^2 weekly for 4 weeks, however, many clinicians use 1 g given twice at a 2 week interval. There appears to be no difference in efficacy between the two regimens. The best maintenance regimen remains to be established with regimens varying between 0.5 and 1 g every 4–6 months for 2 years. Long term use of rituximab is associated with hypogammaglobulinaemia.

4.7.4   Methotrexate

The long-term use of cyclophosphamide is limited due to associated toxicity. In patients with early mild systemic disease, methotrexate with oral steroids is nearly as effective at inducing remission as cyclophosphamide plus oral steroids [9]. For early mild disease or localized disease (this indicates that there is an absence of any threatening organ disease or damage) treatment, methotrexate may be given at a dose of 15 mg/week escalating to a maximum of 20–25 mg/week by week 12 with oral glucocorticoids. However, methotrexate therapy is associated with an increased relapse rate and increased risk of progression to more widespread disease than cyclophosphamide. Methotrexate is excreted via the kidneys and should be used with increased caution in those with serum creatinine >150 µmol/L due to increased toxicity.

Localized disease may have severe local consequences (especially retro-orbital disease) and such patients should receive cyclophosphamide.

4.7.5   Azathioprine

Azathioprine remains the remission maintenance agent of choice. It is associated with intolerance in 5–7 % of cases. The dose of 2 mg/kg/day should be continued for a minimum of 12–18 months before being gradually withdrawn.

4.7.6   Plasma Exchange

Patients presenting with renal failure have much poorer outcomes. A recent trial compared plasma exchange and pulsed methylprednisolone as adjunctive therapy in biopsy-proven AAV with acute renal failure (creatinine >500 µmol/L). Renal outcome was better in the plasma exchange-treated group when expressed as dialysis independence in surviving patients or as overall rate of dialysis-free survival. Death rates were similar in the groups. These results were maintained at 1-year follow-up. Therefore, the addition of plasma exchange to standard treatment regimes improves renal survival but does not affect immediate mortality [10]. Treatment with plasma exchange should be considered in those with other life-threatening manifestations of vasculitis such as pulmonary hemorrhage.

4.8   Monitoring

Careful assessment of these patients to differentiate activity from damage and to consider differential diagnoses is required. Previously unaffected organ systems may be affected many years after the remission is achieved. Patients may develop complication from treatment many years after discontinuation of therapy. Long-term follow-up is necessary for all patients with vasculitis and patients should have rapid access to specialist services.

It is important that a structured clinical assessment is conducted in all patients with vasculitis. This examination may be facilitated by the use of clinical tools that form a checklist of common items affecting various systems in vasculitis, where appropriate scoring systems should be used. A number of scoring systems are available. The Birmingham vasculitis activity score is widely used in clinical trials. Active uncontrolled disease is associated with cumulative organ damage, which should be assessed using the Birmingham vasculitis damage index (see Chap. 3). General health function can be assessed using the SF-36 or HAQ.

This structured examination should be carried out at each clinic visit to detect new organ involvement, which may develop at any time in the disease course. Urine analysis should be performed on each patient at each visit to screen for infection, renal relapse, or response, as well as bladder complications, in patients treated with cyclophosphamide. Inflammatory markers and renal functions should be performed periodically (every 1–3 months) to monitor disease activity and response.

4.9 Patient Advice

The potentially serious complications of the disease and the need for immunosuppressive therapy should be clearly explained.

Attention to the primary prevention of cardiovascular risk should be made; in particular, the treatment of hypertension and hypercholesterolemia. Advice on smoking cessation, healthy diet, and regular exercise should be given.

4.10   Detection and Prevention of the Adverse Effects of Therapy

Treatment for systemic vasculitis often requires high-dose glucocorticoids, cyclophosphamide, or other immunosuppressive agents, which are associated with potential toxicity. This toxicity can be ameliorated with appropriate prophylaxis.

4.10.1   Osteoporosis

All patients receiving corticosteroids for the treatment of vasculitis should be started on a bisphosphonate with calcium and vitamin D supplementation following local guidelines.

4.10.2   Vaccinations

Immunocompromised patients should not receive live vaccines. Patients should receive influenza and pneumococcal vaccinations prior to treatment if possible.

4.10.3   Pneumocystis Jirovecii Infection

Immunosuppressed patients are at risk of *Pneumocystis jiroveci*. There are no RCT data, but observational data support the approach that patients receiving cyclophosphamide and glucocorticoids should receive trimethoprim/sulfamethoxazole 960 mg thrice weekly (or aerolized pentamidine/daily dapsone in patients allergic to trimethoprim/sulfamethoxazole) as prophylaxis against pneumocystis infection.

4.10.4   Cyclophosphamide-Induced Bladder Toxicity

Hemorrhagic cystitis and bladder cancer are recognized complications of therapy. The risk is associated to the cumulative dose of cyclophosphamide administered. Treatment with sodium-2-mercaptoethanesulfonate (MESNA), which protects against the uroepithelial toxicity should be considered in all patients receiving IV cyclophosphamide.

> **Key Points**
> - Treatment of vasculitis depends on the size of the vessel involved and the severity of organ involvement.
> - ANCA-associated vasculitis requires treatment with glucocorticoids and cyclophosphamide depending on disease severity.
> - Intravenous cyclophosphamide is as effective as, and safer than, continuous oral cyclophosphamide.

References

1. Ntatsaki E, Carruthers D, Chakravarty K, et al. BSR/BHPR guideline for the management of adults with ANCA-associated vasculitis. Rheumatology. 2014;53(12):2306–9.
2. Mukhtyar C, Guillevin L, Cid M, et al. EULAR recommendations for the management of large vessel vasculitis. Ann Rheum Dis. 2009;68:318–23.
3. Mukhtyar C, Guillevin L, Cid M, et al. EULAR recommendations for the management of primary small and medium vasculitis. Ann Rheum Dis. 2009;68:310–7.
4. Jayne D, Rasmussen N, Andrassy K, et al. A randomised trial of maintenance therapy for vasculitis associated with antineutrophil cytoplasmic auto antibodies. N Engl J Med. 2003;349:36–44.
5. Pagnoux C, et al. Azathioprine or methotrexate maintenance for ANCA-associated vasculitis. N Engl J Med. 2008;359:2790–803.
6. de Groot K, Harper L, Jayne DR, et al. Pulse versus oral cyclophosphamide for induction of remission in anti-neutrophil cytoplasmic antibody associated vasculitis: a randomised trial. Ann Intern Med. 2009;150:670–80.
7. Jones RB, Tervaert JW, Hauser T, et al. Rituximab versus cyclophosphamide in ANCA-associated renal vasculitis. N Engl J Med. 2010;363:211–20.

8. Stone JH, Merkel PA, Spiera R, et al. Rituximab versus cyclo-phosphamide for ANCA-associated vasculitis. N Engl J Med. 2010;363:221–32.
9. de Groot K, Rasmussen N, Bacon P, et al. Randomised trial of cyclophosphamide versus methotrexate for induction of remission in early systemic antineutrophil cytoplasmic antibody associated vasculitis. Arthritis Rheum. 2005;52:2462–8.
10. Jayne DR, Gaskin G, Rasmussen N, et al. Randomised trial of plasma exchange and high-dosage methylprednisolone as adjunctive therapy for severe renal vasculitis. J Am Soc Nephrol. 2007;18:2180–8.

Part II
Features of Individual Diseases

Chapter 5
Giant Cell Arteritis

5.1 Introduction

Giant cell arteritis (GCA) is the most common systemic vasculitis in the elderly. It is characterized by the involvement of the large vessels, predominantly the extracranial branches of the aorta. There is a close relationship with polymyalgia rheumatica (PMR). The first description of GCA was provided by Sir Jonathon Hutchinson in 1890, who described a patient at the London Hospital who could not wear a hat because of painful red streaks on his head. The painful streaks were thickened temporal arteries with feeble pulsations. The full description of the condition was provided by Bayard Horton in 1932.

5.2 Definition and Classification

The 2012 Chapel Hill Consensus conference defined GCA as "Arteritis, often granulomatous, usually affecting the aorta and/or its major branches, with a predilection for the branches of the carotid and vertebral arteries. Often involves the temporal artery. Onset usually in patients older than 50 years and often associated with polymyalgia rheumatica" [1].

Electronic supplementary material The ownline version of this chapter (doi:10.1007/978-3-319-14871-7_5) contains supplementary material, which is available to authorized users.

R.A. Watts et al., *Vasculitis in Clinical Practice*, DOI 10.1007/978-3-319-14871-7_5,

TABLE 5.1 ACR criteria for the classification of GCA

Age at onset >50 years
Development of symptoms or findings beginning at 50 years or older
New headache
New onset of, or new type of, localized pain in the head
Temporal artery abnormality
Temporal artery tenderness to palpation or decreased pulsation, unrelated to atherosclerosis of the cervical arteries
Increase in erythrocyte sedimentation rate (ESR)
ESR >50 mm/h by Westergren method
Abnormal artery biopsy
Biopsy specimen with an artery showing vasculitis characterized by a predominance of mononuclear infiltration or granulomatous inflammation

From Hunder et al. [2]. With permission from John Wiley and Sons

The ACR in 1990 developed a classification criteria, which are widely used in clinical trials (Table 5.1). A classification of GCA requires three of the five criteria. They have a specificity of 91.2 % and sensitivity of 93.5 % [2]. There are no validated diagnostic criteria.

5.3   Epidemiology

GCA is more common among people of north European descent than among Mediterranean people and is rare among African Americans, native Americans, and Asians. GCA occurs in individuals older than 50 years and the age-adjusted (>50) annual incidence in the UK is 22/100,000 population [3]. The annual incidence rates per 100,000 population rises from 2 in the sixth decade to 52 in the ninth decade [4].

The estimated prevalence is about 1:750 persons older than 50 years. There is a female preponderance; women are two to three times more commonly affected.

5.4   Etiology

The etiology is unknown. There is an association with HLA DRB*0401. Although infectious triggers have long been suspected, no clear associations have yet been confirmed. A proposed hypothesis suggests that the arterial wall dendritic cells become activated and then recruit CD4+ lymphocytes, which become clonally expanded producing IL-2 and IFN-γ. Macrophages produce PDGF, which stimulates intimal arterial thickening. Subsequently, monocyte and macrophages become multinucleate giant cells.

5.5   Clinical Features

The onset of symptoms may be abrupt. Some patients may recall the exact date and hour their symptoms started. In most instances, symptoms are insidious and develop gradually over several weeks.

5.5.1   Systemic

Constitutional features, including fever, fatigue, anorexia, weight loss, and depression are present in the majority of patients. Patients may present with pyrexia of unknown origin.

Myalgia and arthralgia with morning stiffness across the shoulder and hip girdle is suggestive of coexistent PMR.

5.5.2   Craniofacial

Headache is the most common symptom occurring in >60 % of patients. It is typically felt over one or both of the temporal areas. Less commonly the headache may be generalized or occipital. Important features of the headache are that it is different in nature from previous headaches, can be severe or paroxysmal, and be associated with scalp tenderness. Wearing a hat or glasses or combing the hair may be uncomfortable. In severe cases, involvement of the scalp arteries may lead to segmental scalp necrosis (Fig. 5.1).

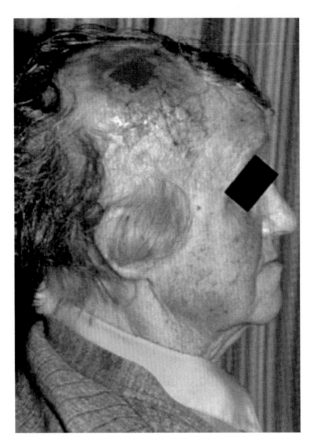

FIGURE 5.1 Scalp necrosis in a patient with giant cell arteritis

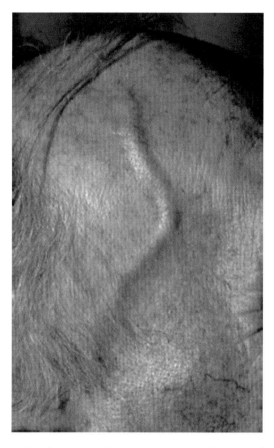

FIGURE 5.2 Swollen temporal artery in a patient with giant cell arteritis

Jaw claudication (30 %), pain in the tongue or jaw during mastication, which resolves with rest may be a risk factor for neuro-ophthalmic complications. In rare cases tongue infarction may result from ischemia.

The temporal arteries may be tender nonpulstaile and thickened (Fig. 5.2). Bruits may be audible over affected arteries especially in the axillae.

5.5.3   Ophthalmic

Ophthalmic manifestations are common and may result in blindness. Acute visual loss occurs in as many as 20 % of patients. The visual loss is usually sudden, painless, and permanent. Visual disturbance may vary from mistiness of vision or involvement of part of the visual field to complete blindness. Visual loss may be bilateral. There may be premonitory symptoms such as blurry vision, amaurosis fugax, visual hallucinations, and diplopia in up to 50 % of cases. These premonitory signs may precede visual loss by several days and should be considered a medical emergency in GCA, as prompt treatment may prevent the development of irreversible blindness.

There are a number of ocular lesions caused by the occlusion of orbital or ocular arteries. Anterior ischemic optic neuropathy is the most common cause of blindness in GCA. Less common causes of visual loss include central retinal artery occlusion, posterior ischemic optic neuropathy, and cortical blindness.

5.5.4   Neurologic

Cerebrovascular ischemic events are uncommon in GCA, occurring in about 3–7 % of GCA patients. Involvement of the vertebrobasilar system is relatively more common in GCA-related CVA than atherosclerotic CVA. Dementia, psychotic features, and depression may occur, but are more likely to be related to high dose corticosteroid therapy.

5.5.5   Extracranial Artery

Extracranial arterial involvement is widespread, especially involving axillary, subclavian, and aortic areas [5, 6]. A careful clinical examination of the arterial tree looking for bruits or weak/absent pulses is essential.

5.6   Laboratory Features

Erythrocyte sedimentation rate (ESR) and C-reactive protein (CRP) are usually significantly increased. The inflammatory markers are normal in <1 % of cases [7]. A normal ESR and CRP does not exclude the diagnosis, but should always prompt a search for a different diagnosis. ESR and CRP can be a useful guide to disease activity, but can be normal in relapse, particularly, if the patient is on glucocorticoids.

Mild to moderate normocytic anemia is observed in 50–70 %. Thrombocytosis and leucocytosis are less commonly seen. Abnormalities of liver function test are recognized with alkaline phosphatase most commonly elevated.

5.6.1   Immunology

Immunology tests such as ANCA, ANA RF, and anticardiolipin antibodies are usually negative.

5.6.2   Imaging

Colour doppler ultrasonography of the temporal and axillary arteries show a characteristic halo sign (Fig. 5.3a, b) (Video 5.1) in active disease which reverses with corticosteroid therapy within 7–10 days.

^{18}FDG-PET scintigraphy is a useful method of assessing disease activity of the aorta and its major branches; however, the temporal arteries cannot be visualized by this method. At present, ^{18}FDG-PET appears to be most useful in the diagnosis of patients presenting with an ill-defined systemic illness, in whom the demonstration of inflammation in large vessels may permit a diagnosis. Its use in the assessment of relapse or remission remains to be determined.

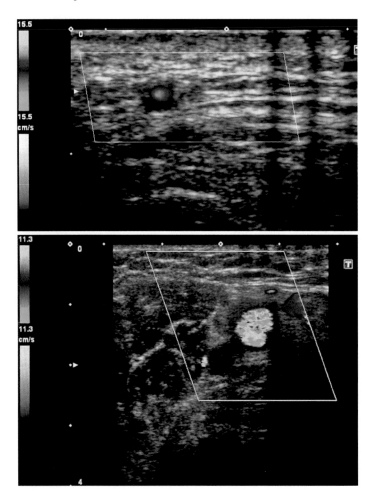

FIGURE 5.3 **a** (*top*) Hypoechoic 'halo' around the temporal artery and **b** (*bottom*) axillary artery

5.6.3   Pathology

A biopsy of the affected temporal artery should be obtained where possible. Histopathological evidence is the gold standard for the diagnosis of giant cell arteritis.

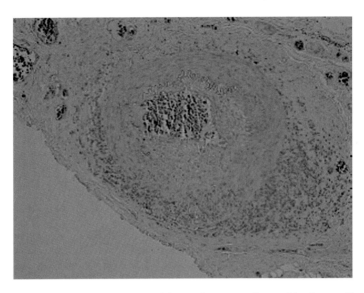

FIGURE 5.4 Temporal artery biopsy from a patient with giant cell arteritis, showing segmental inflammation, including lymphocytes, histiocytes and multinucleated giant cells, of the arterial wall, centered on the internal elastic lamina

There is an inflammatory infiltrate with transmural lymphocytes and macrophages. The internal elastic lamina becomes fragmented and is surrounded by inflammation. Calcific foci may be present. Multinucleated giant cells are often present adjacent to the disrupted internal elastic lamina. The presence of giant cells is not required for the diagnosis if the other typical features are present (Fig. 5.4). A negative biopsy does not exclude the diagnosis, because the lesions are focal in nature and may be missed due to sampling error. An adequate sample length of 1 cm is advised. Routine biopsy of both the temporal arteries is not recommended,. Due to the possibility of a false negative result, and the risk of irreversible ocular involvement, treatment with high-dose glucocorticoids should be commenced on strong clinical suspicion of giant cell arteritis, prior to the biopsy being carried out. Treatment prior to biopsy does not affect the result, provided the biopsy is performed within 2 weeks of initiating glucocorticoid therapy.

5.7   Diagnosis

Raised inflammatory markers are highly sensitive for the diagnosis of giant cell arteritis. A normal ESR or CRP should raise suspicion for an alternative diagnosis, but does not exclude the diagnosis.

The main differential diagnosis is from other causes of a large vessel vasculitis such as Takayasu arteritis. GCA presents at an older age than Takayasu arteritis, which typically presents at age less than 40 years.

Occasionally, patients present with a nonspecific systemic illness, pyrexia of unknown origin, and unexplained anemia, and the differential then includes occult infection and malignancy.

5.8   Assessment of Disease Activity

There are no valid biomarkers for assessing the response and diagnosing the relapse in giant cell arteritis. Clinical monitoring aided by inflammatory markers should guide treatment. A relapse is usually associated with a rise in ESR and CRP. In symptomatic patients, the presence of normal inflammatory markers should raise suspicion of an alternative diagnosis.

5.9   Treatment

Guidelines for the management of GCA have been developed by BSR [8] and EULAR [9]. The general principles have been described in Chap. 4. Early intensive therapy with high-dose glucocorticoid induces remission in patients with giant cell arteritis. Visual loss in one eye is present in 18 % of patients at diagnosis. It is usually irreversible but pulsed intravenous methylprednisolone has been traditionally used to prevent extension of visual loss.. The initial dose of prednisolone is usually 1 mg/kg/day (maximum 60 mg/day) and the initial high-dose glucocorticoid should be maintained for a month and tapered gradually. The taper should not be in the form of alternate day therapy, as this is more likely to lead to a relapse of vasculitis.. The usual duration of glucocorticoid therapy for patients with giant cell arteritis is about 2 years [10]. Some patients may not be able to tolerate complete discontinuation of glucocorticoid therapy due to recurrent disease or secondary adrenal insufficiency. All patients should have bone protection therapy in the absence of contraindications in accordance with local guidelines.

Methotrexate (10–15 mg/week) reduces the relapse rate and lowers the cumulative dose of glucocorticoid therapy [11].

Patients in clinical remission who have discontinued therapy and experience a relapse should be treated as per new patients. For those still on glucocorticoid, an increase of 5–10 mg/day may be sufficient to treat the relapse. Increase to a full remission induction dose of glucocorticoid (1 mg/kg/day) is usually not necessary unless ocular or neurological symptoms recur. Visual loss while taking glucocorticoids is very uncommon.

Patients with giant cell arteritis are at an increased risk of developing cardiovascular and cerebrovascular events and low-dose daily aspirin is usually prescribed.

5.10 Prognosis

Untreated GCA is associated with a significant risk of permanent blindness. This is greatly reduced by the early introduction of corticosteroids. The risk of the second eye being involved in a patient with profound visual loss is 70 % within 1 week unless treated. The risk of blindness in patients on corticosteroids is very low. Life expectancy is not diminished in GCA. Drug toxicity is related to cumulative glucocorticoid use (see Chap. 4).

Key Points

- GCA is the commonest vasculitis affecting the elderly and is commonly accompanied by PMR.
- Typical symptoms include headache, jaw claudication scalp tenderness, visual disturbances, and constitutional symptoms.
- Early recognition and treatment with glucocorticoids can prevent blindness and other complications resulting from occlusion or rupture of the involved arteries.

References

1. Jennette JC, Falk RJ, Bacon PA, Basu N, Cid MC, Ferrario F, et al. 2012 revised International Chapel Hill Consensus Conference Nomenclature of Vasculitides. Arthritis Rheum. 2013;65(1):1–11.
2. Hunder GG, Bloch DA, Michel BA, Stevens MB, Arend WP, Calabrese LH, et al. The American College of Rheumatology 1990 criteria for the classification of giant cell arteritis. Arthritis Rheum. 1990;33(8):1122–8.
3. Smeeth L, Cook C, Hall AJ. Incidence of diagnosed polymyalgia rheumatica and temporal arteritis in the United Kingdom, 1990–2001. Ann Rheum Dis. 2006;65(8):1093–8.
4. Salvarani C, Gabriel SE, O'Fallon WM, Hunder GG. The incidence of giant cell arteritis in Olmsted County, Minnesota: apparent fluctuations in a cyclic pattern. Ann Intern Med. 1995;123(3):192–4.
5. Blockmans D, de Ceuninck L, Vanderschueren S, Knockaert D, Mortelmans L, Bobbaers H. Repetitive 18F-fluorodeoxyglucose positron emission tomography in giant cell arteritis: a prospective study of 35 patients. Arthritis Rheum. 2006;55(1):131–7.
6. Schmidt WA, Seifert A, Gromnica-Ihle E, Krause A, Natusch A. Ultrasound of proximal upper extremity arteries to increase the diagnostic yield in large-vessel giant cell arteritis. Rheumatology (Oxford). 2008;47(1):96–101.
7. Parikh M, Miller NR, Lee AG, Savino PJ, Vacarezza MN, Cornblath W, et al. Prevalence of a normal C-reactive protein with an elevated erythrocyte sedimentation rate in biopsy-proven giant cell arteritis. Ophthalmology. 2006;113(10):1842–5.

8. Dasgupta B, Borg FA, Hassan N, Alexander L, Barraclough K, Bourke B, et al. BSR and BHPR guidelines for the management of giant cell arteritis. Rheumatology (Oxford). 2010;49(8): 1594–7.

9. Mukhtyar C, Guillevin L, Cid MC, Dasgupta B, de Groot K, Gross W, et al. EULAR recommendations for the management of large vessel vasculitis. Ann Rheum Dis. 2009;68(3):318–23.

10. Proven A, Gabriel SE, Orces C, O'Fallon WM, Hunder GG. Glucocorticoid therapy in giant cell arteritis: duration and adverse outcomes. Arthritis Rheum. 2003;49(5):703–8.

11. Mahr AD, Jover JA, Spiera RF, Hernandez-Garcia C, Fernandez-Gutierrez B, Lavalley MP, et al. Adjunctive methotrexate for treatment of giant cell arteritis: an individual patient data meta-analysis. Arthritis Rheum. 2007;56(8):2789–97.

Chapter 6
Takayasu Arteritis

6.1 Introduction

Takayasu arteritis (TA) is a granulomatous vasculitis of unknown etiology occurring in young people and is characterized by stenosis, occlusion, and sometimes aneurysm formation of large arteries. TA has various names including pulseless disease, aortic arch syndrome, long-segment atypical coarctation of the aorta, Martorell's syndrome, and occlusive thromboaortopathy. The first full description of the natural history and pathology of Takayasu arteritis was provided by Sir William Savory in 1856. He described a 13 month in-patient stay of a 22 year old woman with obliteration of the carotid and subclavian arteries. He attributed the autopsy appearances of the arteries to an inflammatory condition [1].

6.2 Definition and Classification

The Chapel Hill consensus conference defined TA as "Arteritis, often granulomatous, predominantly affectingthe aorta and/or its major branches. Onset usually in patients younger than 50 years" [2].

The ACR in 1990 developed the classification criteria which are widely used in clinical trials. The presence of any three or more criteria yields a sensitivity of 90.5 % and specificity of 97.8 % [2] (Table 6.1).

R.A. Watts et al., *Vasculitis in Clinical Practice*,
DOI 10.1007/978-3-319-14871-7_6,
© Springer International Publishing AG, Cham 2015

TABLE 6.1 ACR classification criteria for TA

Age <40 years old
Development of symptoms or signs related to TA at age <40 years
Claudication of extremities
Development and worsening of fatigue and discomfort in muscles of one or more extremity while in use, especially the upper extremities
Decreased brachial arterial pulse
Decreased pulsation of one or both brachial arteries
BP difference >10 mmHg
Difference of >10 mmHg in systolic blood pressure between arms
Bruit over subclavian arteries or aorta
Bruit audible on auscultation over one or both subclavian arteries or abdominal aorta
Arteriogram abnormality
Arteriographic narrowing or occlusion of the entire aorta, its proximal branches, or large arteries in the proximal upper or lower extremities, not due to atherosclerosis, fibromuscular dysplasia, or similar causes; changes usually focal or segmental

From Arend et al. [3] With permission from John Wiley and Sons

6.3   Epidemiology

TA occurs throughout the world and may have a varying clinical spectrum in different populations. TA is believed to be predominantly found in Asia, the Middle East and South America. Patients with TA have been increasingly recognized in Africa, Europe, and North America. The incidence in Europe and USA is 0.5–2.5/million/year [4–6]. In Japan, the incidence is probably much higher. In an autopsy study, Hotchi describes the frequency of TA in 0.033 % of all autopsies [7]. Most series report a female preponderance. Symptom onset is typically aged less than 40 years, with a median age of onset 25–30 years.

6.4   Etiology

The strong racial distribution of the disease may be genetic, but it does not have to be. Although, familial forms of TA have been described, the disease does not have strong inheritance. IL12B region on chromosome 5, MLX region on chromosome 17, and HLA-B*52:01 have been shown to be significant associations for TA [8]. IL12B region seems to play an important part in the pathophysiology. It exhibits a synergistic effect when co-present with HLA-B*52:01 in increasing the risk of TA. IL12B region also demonstrates an association with aortic regurgitation in TA [8]. The IL12B association has been verified in a separate multi-ethnic cohort [9]. Two additional HLA susceptibility loci have been identified at HLA-DQB1/HLA-DRB1 and HLA-B/MICA [9].

6.5   Clinical Features

6.5.1   Systemic

Systemic symptoms may be present in up to 20–40 % of patients and include fatigue weight loss, night sweats, fever, arthralgia, and myalgia.

6.5.2   Vascular

At the time of diagnosis, approximately 20 % of patients with TA have no vascular symptoms, with the disease being detected by abnormal clinical findings. The most common findings at presentation are absence or asymmetry of peripheral pulses, claudication of arm or legs, transient visual disturbance, scotoma, blurring, or diplopia.

On physical examination, the most common features are diminished or absent pulses, bruits, and asymmetric blood pressure measurements between extremities. Carotidynia (tenderness of the carotid arteries) is rare but characteristic. Hypertension occurs in approximately 28 % of patients with TA and is due to coarctation of the aorta or renal artery stenosis.

6.6   Laboratory Features

The most common laboratory finding is the presence of elevated inflammatory markers (ESR and/or CRP) and a blood picture reflective of acute inflammation. There may be a normochromic normocytic anemia with leukocytosis and thrombocytosis.

6.6.1   Immunology

TA is not associated with the presence of ANCA, RF, ANA, and anticardiolipin antibodies.

6.6.2   Imaging

Since 2004, there have been several case series demonstrating the utility of physiological imaging in the form of 18-fluorodeoxyglucose (FDG) labeled positron emission tomography (PET) (Fig. 6.1) [10]. The advantage of this modality over conventional computed tomography (CT) or magnetic resonance (MR) angiography is its ability to demonstrate intramural inflammation which precedes luminal changes. PET-CT scanning is now the accepted modality for the diagnosis of TA. However the radiation exposure of approximately 25 mSv and the inability of the modality to correlate with disease activity mean that it is not a good modality for monitoring of disease activity.

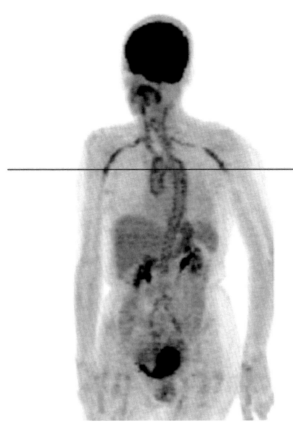

FIGURE 6.1 ^{18}F-fluorodeoxyglucose positron emission tomography (^{18}F-FDG-PET) in a patient with TA showing increased up take of ^{18}F-FDG in the aorta and subclavian vessels

Magnetic resonance angiography can provide high-resolution imaging of the anatomical features including mural thickening, luminal changes, and wall enhancement (Fig. 6.2). The combination of these changes could provide additional information for assessing disease activity, and therefore this becomes a safe modality for monitoring [11].

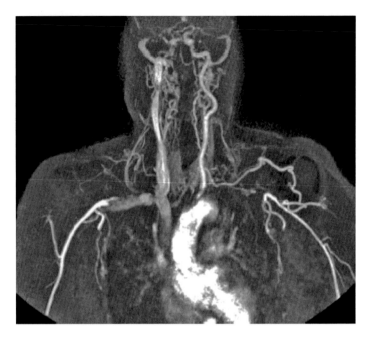

FIGURE 6.2 Magnetic resonance angiography in patient with Takayasu arteritis (TA) showing narrowing of subclavian vessels bilaterally and the left internal carotid together with development of a collateral circulation

Digital subtraction angiography, CT angiography and Ultrasonography are occasionally useful in the presence of contraindication to MRA.

6.6.3   Pathology

The appearances are of a granulomatous necrotizing vasculitis affecting large vessels. In the acute inflammatory phase there is adventitial thickening, cellular infiltration of the tunica media, with local destruction of the vascular smooth muscle. The intima becomes fibrosed, which leads to vessel stenosis.

6.7   Diagnosis

The diagnosis of TA is based on the demonstration of vascular inflammation in large and middle-sized vessels on PET-CT scanning, or structural changes by other forms of imaging. The differential diagnosis includes giant cell arteritis and IgG4 related disease. GCA typically occurs after 60 years of age. The vascular involvement of IgG4 is patchy, less likely to be stenotic, and more likely to be associated with hepatobiliary, pancreatic, or retroperitoneal involvement.

6.8   Assessment of Disease Activity

Although inflammatory markers are typically raised, ESR has not been consistently shown to be a good marker for active inflammatory disease. Some patients have progressive disease with normal inflammatory markers. MR Angiography is useful to monitor disease progression. There is limited evidence for the use of carotid and subclavian ultrasonography for monitoring TA. All the imaging modalities need formal validation for monitoring vasculitis activity.

6.9   Treatment

Guidelines for the management of large vessel vasculitis have been developed by EULAR [12].

6.9.1   Pharmacological Therapy

It is recognized that early intensive therapy induces remission in TA. Treatment involves high-dose oral prednisolone at 0.5–1 mg/kg (maximum 60 mg). The dose should be tapered aiming for 10 mg/day at 6 months. Despite glucocorticoid therapy, TA can remain active at a subclinical level. There is some evidence for the use of Azathioprine (2 mg/kg/day) as an adjunct to glucocorticoid therapy [13]. In cases of refractory disease there is some evidence for the use of biologic therapies such as TNF blockade [14] and IL-6 antagonists [15].

6.9.2   Surgery

Surgical intervention is indicated for severe ischemic organ involvement as established stenotic lesions are not reversible with medical treatment alone. Surgical procedures include bypass grafting and percutaneous procedures including angioplasty and intraluminal stenting. Surgical treatment is indicated in patients with severe complications of TA, particularly cerebrovascular disease due to cervicocranial stenosis, coronary artery disease, severe to moderate aortic insufficiency, severe coarctation of the aorta, renovascular hypertension, limb claudication, and progressive aneurysm enlargement. Revascularization should only be considered if stenotic or occlusive lesions are leading to aneurysmal lesions which may rupture. There is a high restenosis rate of 20–30 %. In general, bypass grafting is less prone to restenosis compared to stent placement [16]. Elective procedures should be performed when the disease is in remission.

6.10   Prognosis

The overall mortality rate is low at around 3 % in the USA. However, the long-term outcome has varied between studies. Mortality directly related to TA usually occurs from congestive cardiac failure, cerebrovascular events, myocardial infarction, aneurysm rupture, or renal failure. There is a high prevalence of metabolic syndrome in TA [17]. Relapse is common (96 %) [18].

Key Points

- Takayasu arteritis (TA) is a granulomatous vasculitis of unknown etiology, characterized by stenosis, occlusion, and sometimes aneurysm formation of large arteries.
- The most common findings at presentation are absence or asymmetry of peripheral pulses, claudication of arm or legs, transient visual disturbance scotoma, blurring, or diplopia.
- PET-CT scanning is useful for diagnosis of TA, and MRA is useful for monitoring of disease.

References

1. Savory WS. Case of a Young Woman in whom the main Arteries of both Upper Extremities and of the Left Side of the Neck were throughout completely Obliterated. Med Chir Trans. 1856;39:205–19.
2. Jennette JC, Falk RJ, Bacon PA, Basu N, Cid MC, Ferrario F, et al. 2012 revised International Chapel Hill Consensus Conference Nomenclature of Vasculitides. Arthritis Rheum. 2013;65(1):1–11.
3. Arend WP, Michel BA, Bloch DA, Hunder GG, Calabrese LH, Edworthy SM, et al. The American College of Rheumatology 1990 criteria for the classification of Takayasu arteritis. Arthritis Rheum. 1990;33(8):1129–34.
4. Dreyer L, Faurschou M, Baslund B. A population-based study of Takayasu s arteritis in eastern Denmark. Clin Exp Rheumatol. 2011;29(1 Suppl 64):S40–2.
5. Hall S, Barr W, Lie JT, Stanson AW, Kazmier FJ, Hunder GG. Takayasu arteritis. A study of 32 North American patients. Medicine (Baltimore). 1985;64(2):89–99.
6. Watts R, Al-Taiar A, Mooney J, Scott D, Macgregor A. The epidemiology of Takayasu arteritis in the UK. Rheumatology (Oxford). 2009;48(8):1008–11.
7. Hotchi M. Pathological studies on Takayasu arteritis. Heart Vessels Suppl. 1992;7:11–7.

8. Terao C, Yoshifuji H, Kimura A, Matsumura T, Ohmura K, Takahashi M, et al. Two susceptibility loci to Takayasu arteritis reveal a synergistic role of the IL12B and HLA-B regions in a Japanese population. Am J Hum Genet. 2013;93(2):289–97.

9. Saruhan-Direskeneli G, Hughes T, Aksu K, Keser G, Coit P, Aydin SZ, et al. Identification of multiple genetic susceptibility loci in Takayasu arteritis. Am J Hum Genet. 2013;93(2):298–305.

10. de Leeuw K, Bijl M, Jager PL. Additional value of positron emission tomography in diagnosis and follow-up of patients with large vessel vasculitides. Clin Exp Rheumatol. 2004;22(6 Suppl 36):S21–6.

11. Jiang L, Li D, Yan F, Dai X, Li Y, Ma L. Evaluation of Takayasu arteritis activity by delayed contrast-enhanced magnetic resonance imaging. Int J Cardiol. 2012;155(2):262–7.

12. Mukhtyar C, Guillevin L, Cid MC, Dasgupta B, de Groot K, Gross W, et al. EULAR recommendations for the management of large vessel vasculitis. Ann Rheum Dis. 2009;68(3):318–23.

13. Valsakumar AK, Valappil UC, Jorapur V, Garg N, Nityanand S, Sinha N. Role of immunosuppressive therapy on clinical, immunological, and angiographic outcome in active Takayasu's arteritis. J Rheumatol. 2003;30(8):1793–8.

14. Hoffman GS, Merkel PA, Brasington RD, Lenschow DJ, Liang P. Anti-tumor necrosis factor therapy in patients with difficult to treat Takayasu arteritis. Arthritis Rheum. 2004;50(7):2296–304.

15. Tombetti E, Franchini S, Papa M, Sabbadini MG, Baldissera E. Treatment of refractory Takayasu arteritis with tocilizumab: 7 Italian patients from a single referral center. J Rheumatol. 2013;40(12):2047–51.

16. Lee GY, Jeon P, Do YS, Sung K, Kim DI, Kim YW, et al. Comparison of outcomes between endovascular treatment and bypass surgery in Takayasu arteritis. Scand J Rheumatol. 2014;43(2):153–61.

17. da Silva TF, Levy-Neto M, Bonfa E, Pereira RM. High prevalence of metabolic syndrome in Takayasu arteritis: increased cardiovascular risk and lower adiponectin serum levels. J Rheumatol. 2013;40(11):1897–904.

18. Maksimowicz-McKinnon K, Clark TM, Hoffman GS. Limitations of therapy and a guarded prognosis in an American cohort of Takayasu arteritis patients. Arthritis Rheum. 2007;56(3):1000–9.

Chapter 7
Granulomatosis with Polyangiitis – GPA (Wegeners)

7.1 Introduction

GPA is a rare form of systemic vasculitis of unknown etiology, characterized by the involvement of the upper airway with granuloma formation and renal involvement with vasculitis. Although attributed to Wegener, it was first described by Klinger in 1931.

7.2 Definition and Classification

The Chapel Hill Consensus Conference defined GPA as "Necrotizing granulomatous inflammation usually involving the upper and lower respiratory tract, and necrotizing vasculitis affecting predominantly small to medium vessels (e.g., capillaries, venules, arterioles, arteries and veins). Necrotizing glomerulonephritis is common" [1]. It is also very often associated with ANCA, usually of PR3 specificity.

The usual criteria used for classifying GPA are those of the ACR (Table 7.1). For purposes of classification, a person is said to have GPA if at least two of these four criteria are present. The presence of any two or more yields a sensitivity of 88.2 % and a specificity of 92 % [2].

R.A. Watts et al., *Vasculitis in Clinical Practice*,
DOI 10.1007/978-3-319-14871-7_7,
© Springer International Publishing AG, Cham 2015

TABLE 7.1 ACR (1990) criteria for the classification of GPA (Wegener's)

Nasal or oral inflammation
Development of painful or painless oral ulcers or purulent or bloody nasal discharge
Abnormal chest radiograph
Chest radiograph showing the presence of nodules, fixed infiltrates or cavities
Urinary sediment
Microhaematuria (>5 red cells per high power field) or red cell casts in urinary sediment
Granulomatous inflammation on biopsy
Histological changes showing granulomatous inflammation within the wall of an artery or in the perivascular or extravascular area (artery or arteriole)

From Leavitt et al. [2] With permission from John Wiley and Sons

7.3 Epidemiology

There are significant variations in the incidence of GPA in different parts of the world. In northern Europe, including the UK, the incidence is approximately 10/million/year and commonest age of onset is between 60 and 70 years, but GPA has been described in all ages, including children and patients in their 90s [3]. GPA appears to be much rarer in southern Europe and in Japan (less than 3/million/year). Its prevalence ranges between 50 and 300 patients/million, with data from the UK suggesting that the prevalence of GPA is approximately 130 patients/million.

7.4 Etiology

The etiology of GPA is unknown. Like many autoimmune diseases, it is generally believed to result from an environmental trigger, such as silica, interacting with a genetically predisposed host. Genetic factors have been extensively studied, but there is an association with HLA-DP. The familial genetic risk is similar to that seen in RA. No infectious triggers have been identified, although incidence figures from Norfolk have shown a periodicity every 7 or so years which is compatible with an infectious etiology. The association with PR3 ANCA suggests a possible role for the antibody in pathogenesis and this has been studied in animal models with inconclusive results. Non-MHC genetic links include associations with PTPN 22 and CTLA4. Recent Genome Wide Association Studies (GWAS) suggest genetic influences reflect the ANCA specificity (PR3 or MPO) more than the phenotype. Environmental factors have also been studied extensively and silica is probably the best documented.

7.5   Clinical Features

GPA often presents with upper airway/ENT manifestations, but can present in a number of different ways, including a severe widespread systemic illness. The prodromal phase, which may last weeks, months, or even years, consists of predominantly ENT symptoms, such as epistaxis, nasal crusting, and sinusitis, and these symptoms, particularly if followed/accompanied by a systemic illness, should alert the physician to the possibility of GPA as a diagnosis.

7.5.1   Systemic

Fever, weight loss, myalgia, and arthralgia are common. Many patients describe a prodromal illness with a constitutional illness.

7.5.2   Pulmonary

Pulmonary symptoms include cough, hemoptysis, and dyspnoea.

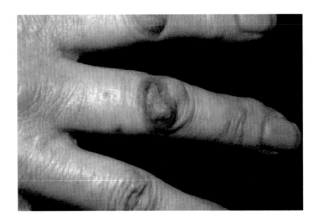

FIGURE 7.1 Skin rash in a patient with GPA

7.5.3   Cutaneous

Skin involvement is seen in 40 % of patients and is most classically a palpable purpura, and histology of such a rash
reveals a leukocytoclastic vasculitis (Fig. 7.1). Cutaneous
ulceration can also occur, as can digital gangrene, but the latter is relatively rare.

7.5.4   ENT

GPA often presents with upper airway/ENT manifestations.
The typical ENT symptoms are epistaxis, nasal crusting, and
sinusitis. Cartilage destruction may lead to nasal collapse
(Fig. 7.2).

7.5.5   Gastrointestinal

Gastrointestinal manifestations are relatively uncommon,
but important to recognize. Abdominal pain, diarrhea, nausea, vomiting, and bleeding can all occur and vasculitis and
granuloma can be found within the GI tract, resulting in small

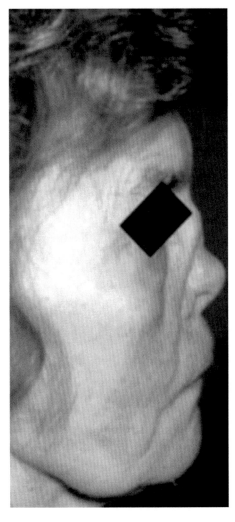

FIGURE 7.2 Nasal bridge collapse in a patient with GPA

bowel ischemia, which can be life-threatening. More common are nonspecific symptoms and evidence of liver dysfunction as assessed by abnormal liver function tests which more probably reflect inflammation (see below).

7.5.6   Neurological

Nervous system involvement is not uncommon and occurs in approximately 20 % of patients. It is, however, much rarer to see overt mononeuritis multiplex in GPA than in EGPA. The most common finding is a mild peripheral sensory neuropathy.

7.5.7   Renal

Renal involvement is very common and the kidney is one of the most important organs to be involved in GPA. The classical features are of indolent onset renal failure and it is vital that all patients with suspected GPA have regular urine checks because the presence of an abnormal sediment, particularly the combination of blood and protein in the urine, is a strong indicator of renal involvement.

7.5.8   Eye

Scleritis is not uncommon (10–20 %), but the most serious ocular complication/involvement associated with GPA is proptosis due to retro-orbital granuloma formation, which can lead to blindness. It is often painful and can be difficult to treat. ENT involvement in the upper airway can be associated with CNS involvement, either due to direct extension through the cribriform plate or from systemic spread, but meningeal enhancement associated with headaches is not infrequent, and specific CNS involvements including inflammation, infarction, and even diabetes insipidus have all been described.

7.5.9   Musculoskeletal

Nonspecific myalgia and arthralgia are common and polyarthritis is well described. GPA can present in an identical way to rheumatoid arthritis with a symmetrical peripheral polyarthritis, so it needs to be considered within that differential diagnosis. Large joint arthritis can also occur, but arthralgia and myalgia are the commonest presenting symptoms.

7.5.10 Cardiac

Cardiac involvement is also well described in GPA, but relatively rare and certainly rarer than in EGPA. Pericarditis, myocarditis, arythmias and myocardial infarction are all recognized problems accompanying GPA.

7.6 Laboratory Features

Investigations are required for assessing the severity/activity of disease and for diagnosis and usually comprise a combination of laboratory, radiological, and histological tests.

Full blood count may show a normochromic, normocytic anemia. White count is usually normal or slightly raised, but leucopaenia is very unusual. The acute phase response is almost always very raised at presentation and inflammatory markers such as ESR and CRP are good indirect measures of disease activity.

Liver function tests are frequently slightly abnormal (especially raised gamma GT and alkaline phosphatase). These most commonly reflect inflammation rather than specific liver involvement, though granulomata and hepatic blood vessel involvement can occur.

7.6.1 Immunology

Immunology tests are very helpful in diagnosis. ANCA is positive in over 90 % of patients with GPA [4]. The majority have c-ANCA (cytoplasmic staining) on indirect immunofluorescence, and when the antigen specificity is tested (as it should be in all cases), it most commonly is associated with PR3.

Other immunology investigations are important as they exclude important differential diagnoses such as antinuclear antibodies (for SLE), rheumatoid factor (for rheumatoid

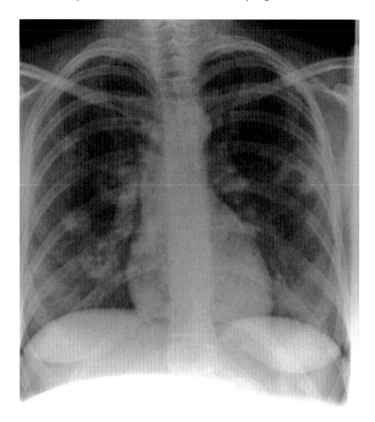

FIGURE 7.3 CXR showing pulmonary nodules in a patient with GPA

arthritis), cryoglobulins (cryoglobulinaemia), anticardiolipin antibodies (for antiphospholipid syndrome), and complement levels. Complement levels are reduced in immune complex vasculitis (Cryoglobulinaemic vasculitis, IgA vasculitis, lupus, etc.), but not in GPA.

7.6.2   Imaging

The chest X-ray or CT thorax in GPA characteristically shows nodular shadowing due to granuloma formation and these nodules may cavitate (Figs. 7.3 and 7.4). These chest

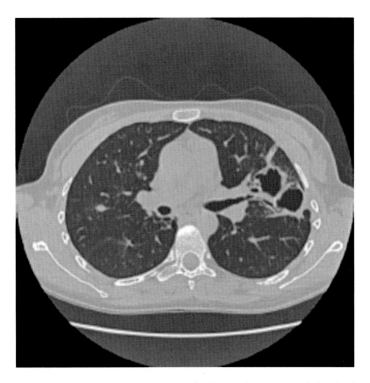

FIGURE 7.4 CT thorax showing cavitating pulmonary nodules in a patient with GPA

features contrast with the fleeting pulmonary infiltrates of EGPA and the pulmonary hemorrhage characteristic of MPA, though pulmonary hemorrhage can occur rarely in GPA.

Cranial MRI is useful for visualizing nasal, sinusoidal, orbital (retrobulbar), and mastoidal lesions (Fig. 7.5) and can be used to guide biopsy.

7.6.3 Pathology

The characteristic pathological features of GPA are granulomatous inflammation, tissue necrosis, and small-medium

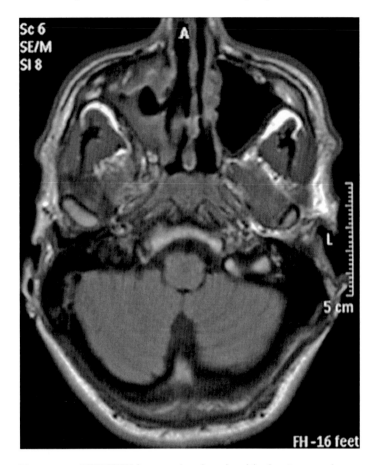

FIGURE 7.5 MRI T1W images showing sinusitis due to granuloma-tous tissue

vessel vasculitis. The full triad of features is found in only one third of pulmonary biopsies. Granulomata may be found in any tissue, but are rarely found in renal biopsies. The renal biopsy characteristically shows a focal segmental necrotizing glomerulonephritis with crescent formation. A skin biopsy shows a leucocytoclastic vasculitis.

7.7   Diagnosis

7.7.1   Differential Diagnosis

The important differential diagnoses are the other systemic vasculitides particularly MPA, EGPA, and polyarteritis nodosa, besides a number of vasculitic mimics including malignancy, cholesterol embolism, atrial myxoma (another reason for echocardiography), and infection. Blood cultures are thus important, as is viral serology because of the association of vasculitis with HBV, HCV, HIV, and CMV. Destructive nasal disease can be associated with substance abuse, particularly cocaine, which also needs to be considered.

7.7.2   Assessment of Organ Involvement

Individual organ involvement should be assessed. Renal function tests are the most important, particularly urinalysis (see above). Urinalysis should be performed urgently in all patients in whom systemic vasculitis is suspected, looking for proteinuria, hematuria, and red cell casts. Renal function may be assessed by creatinine clearance, 24-h urine protein excretion, or protein/creatinine ratios. In the presence of evidence of renal involvement, renal biopsy is important to assess the severity and extent of inflammation with the commonest finding being a focal segmental necrotizing glomerulonephritis, with few if any immune deposits.

Chest X-ray may show granuloma formation and/or hemorrhage. Pulmonary hemorrhage may be confirmed with bronchoalveolar lavage and a raised K_{CO}.

Other investigations are required, depending on clinical involvement. For example, nerve condition studies and neural biopsy can be helpful in the presence of neuropathy. ECG and echocardiography are used to assess cardiac function (echocardiography should be done as a screen with all patients with suspected vasculitis because of the importance of excluding bacterial endocarditis).

With severe gut involvement, angiography may be performed and aneurysms identical to those seen in polyarteritis nodosa are seen in a small minority of patients.

7.8   Assessment of Disease Activity

The most commonly used assessment is the Birmingham Vasculitis Score (BVAS) [5]. Active uncontrolled disease is associated with cumulative organ damage which can be assessed using the Birmingham Vasculitis Damage Index (VDI), and general health function can be assessed using SF-36 or HAQ [5].

Clinical assessment is particularly important in monitoring disease activity and careful monitoring for deterioration in renal function because if disease flares, significant renal involvement can result in irreversible renal damage, renal failure, and a requirement for dialysis. Blood tests such as CRP may be useful for detecting inflammation during assessment and regular urinalysis is vital to pick up early renal involvement. The utility of serial determinations of ANCA to predict relapse, and hence, changes in therapy remains controversial [6]. Overall, low predictive values for relapse were found, so it is not justified to escalate immunosuppressive therapy solely on the basis of an increase in ANCA level, as determined by PR3/MPO ELISA. An increase should be taken as a warning and the patient observed more closely. The aim of therapy is to induce and maintain remission with a minimum of tissue damage due to either disease activity or therapy.

7.9   Treatment

Guidelines on the management of GPA have been recently published [7, 8]. The intensity of initial immunosuppression depends on the severity of organ involvement and size of vessels involved (Table 4.1; Fig. 4.1). Therefore, an important part of treatment planning involves assessment of organ involvement and its severity. Treatment may be divided in to remission induction, maintenance, and long-term follow-up (see Chap. 4 for details).

7.9.1 Remission Induction

Remission induction is usually undertaken using a combination of corticosteroids and cyclophosphamide. Pulse intravenous cyclophosphamide is associated with similar responses to oral cyclophosphamide but fewer side-effects, probably due to lower cumulative dosage. A number of regimens have been described; most use two-weekly intravenous cyclophosphamide, maximum 15 mg/kg (but reduce with renal impairment and age) for three consecutive infusions, thereafter reducing frequency to three weekly for between 3 and 6 months. Mesna may be used to reduce risk of bladder toxicity and intermittent oral septrin is advised for PCP prophylaxis. B cell depletion with Rituximab is an alternative treatment for remission induction [9, 10] and is used when there are concerns for fertility or other contraindications to the use of cyclophosphamide. Rituximab is also often used for relapsing disease as there is evidence that the long term toxicity of cyclophosphamide is closely related to the cumulative doe – the risk being particularly high at cumulative doses over 15 g

7.9.2 Maintenance

Once remission has been induced, oral Azathioprine or Methotrexate is the standard treatment which needs to be given for at least 18 months. In particularly severe disease, plasma exchange needs to be given in addition to the above remission induction therapy.

When Rituximab is used for remission induction or for relapse, there may not be any requirement for additional immunosuppression with these drugs.

7.10   Prognosis

Untreated GPA is associated with a high mortality, which has been substantially improved following the introduction of corticosteroid plus cyclophosphomide as outlined above. With current treatment regimens, the mortality is around 20 % at 5 years [11]. Poor prognostic factors include age over 60 at presentation, severe renal disease, and pulmonary hemorrhage. Long-term follow-up reveals that relapses are not uncommon, with up to 50 % relapsing by 5 years. After the early mortality (usually within 3–6 months), the survival curve follows that of the general population for up to 8–10 years and then appears to increase, probably due to an excess of cardiovascular deaths. Once remission has been induced, it is important thus to address cardiovascular risk factors such as cholesterol, blood pressure, smoking, etc. during long-term follow-up.

Morbidity is also important, particularly for upper airway disease which can be more difficult to control than the systemic vasculitis. Nasal bridge collapse, resulting in deformity and difficulty with breathing, destructive sinus disease resulting in recurrent sinus infections and granulomatous ocular involvement with proptosis are all important features that may need more specialist management and involvement with ENT surgeons and plastic surgeons.

Key Points
- GPA is the commonest of the ANCA-associated vasculitides with an incidence of approximately 10/million/year in northern Europe
- It is frequently associated with the presence of PR3 ANCA
- There is significant variation in the incidence of GPA throughout the world, it being commoner in northern than southern Europe and commoner in Europe than in the far east, including Japan

- Early recognition and treatment are essential to prevent early mortality
- Remission induction is best with intravenous pulse cyclophosphomide and corticosteroids, or with Rituximab
- After remission induction, GPA is managed as a chronic, potentially relapsing disease with careful monitoring and follow-up
- The most difficult systems to treat are those associated with granuloma formation, particularly in the upper airways and in the retro-orbital space

References

1. Jennette JC, Falk RJ, Bacon PA, et al. 2012 Revised international Chapel Hill Consensus Conference nomenclature of vasculitides. Arthritis Rheum. 2013;65:1–11.
2. Leavitt RY, Fauci AS, Bloch DA, et al. The American College of Rheumatology 1990 criteria for the classification of Wegener's granulomatosis. Arthritis Rheum. 1990;33:1101–7.
3. Watts RA, Scott DGI. Epidemiology of vasculitis. In: Ball GV, Bridges L, editors. Vasculitis. 3rd ed. Oxford: Oxford University Press; 2014. p. 7–28.
4. Choi HK, Liu S, Merkel PA, Colditz GA, Niles JL. Diagnostic performance of antineutrophil cytoplasmic antibody tests for idiopathic vasculitides: metaanalysis with a focus on antimyeloperoxidase antibodies. J Rheumatol. 2001;28:1584–90.
5. Luqmani RA. Assessment of vasculitis. In: Ball GV, Bridges L, editors. Vasculitis. 3rd ed. Oxford: Oxford University Press; 2014. p. 299–306.
6. Birck R, Schmitt W, Kaelsch IA, van Der Woude FJ. Serial ANCA determinations for monitoring disease activity in patients with ANCA-associated vasculitis: systematic review. Am J Kidney Dis. 2006;47:15–23.
7. Ntatsaki E, Carruthers D, Chakravarty K, D'Cruz D, Harper L, Jayne DRW, Luqmani RA, Venning M, Mooney J, Mills J, Watts RA. BSR and BHPR guidelines for the management of adults with ANCA associated vasculitis. Rheumatology. 2014;53(1): 145–52.

8. Mukhtyar C, Guillevin L, Cid M, et al. EULAR recommendations for the management of primary small and medium vasculitis. Ann Rheum Dis. 2009;68:310–7.

9. Jones RB, Tervaert JW, Hauser T, et al. Rituximab versus cyclophosphamide in ANCA-associated renal vasculitis. N Engl J Med. 2010;363:211–20.

10. Stone JH, Merkel PA, Spiera R, et al. Rituximab versus cyclophosphamide for ANCA-associated vasculitis. N Engl J Med. 2010;363:221–32.

11. Phillip R, Luqmani R. Mortality in systemic vasculitis: a systematic review. Clin Exp Rheumatol. 2008;26 suppl 5:S94–101.

Chapter 8
Eosinophilic Granulomatosis with Polyangiitis – EGPA (Churg–Strauss Syndrome)

8.1 Introduction

EGPA, also known as allergic granulomatous angiitis, is a rare, anti-neutrophil cytoplasmic antibody (ANCA) associated small vessel vasculitis. It was first described in 1951 by Churg and Strauss and is a multisystem disorder, characterized by allergic rhinitis and asthma, eosinophilia, and extravascular granulomata.

8.2 Definition and Classification

EGPA is defined using the Chapel Hill consensus definitions (2012) "Eosinophil-rich and necrotizing granulomatous inflammation often involving the respiratory tract, and necrotizing vasculitis predominantly affecting small to medium vessels, and associated with asthma and eosinophilia. ANCA is more frequent when glomerulonephritis is present [1]."

There are three main classification schemes for EGPA. The Chapel Hill Consensus Conference definition (above) is based on clinical and histopathological features, Lanham's criteria (Table 8.1) put emphasis on clinical presentation [2] and the ACR criteria (Table 8.2) developed in 1990 [3]. The presence of four or more out of six criteria yields a sensitivity of 85 % and a specificity of 99.7 %.

R.A. Watts et al., *Vasculitis in Clinical Practice*,
DOI 10.1007/978-3-319-14871-7_8,
© Springer International Publishing AG, Cham 2015

TABLE 8.1 Lanham criteria for EGPA

Asthma
Peripheral eosinophilia $>1 \times 10^9$/L
Systemic vasculitis involving two or more extrapulmonary organs

From Lanham et al. [2]

TABLE 8.2 ACR criteria for EGPA

Asthma
  History of wheezing or diffuse high-pitched rales on
    expiration

Eosinophilia
  Greater than 10 % of white blood cell differential count

Mononeuropathy or polyneuropathy
  Development of mononeuropathy, multiple
    mononeuropathies, or polyneuropathy
(i.e., glove/stocking distribution) attributable to vasculitis

Pulmonary infiltrates, nonfixed
  Migratory or transitory pulmonary infiltrates on radiographs
    (not including fixed infiltrates), attributable to systemic
    vasculitis

Paranasal sinus abnormality
  History of acute or chronic paranasal sinus pain or tenderness
    or radiographic opacification of the paranasal sinuses

Extravascular eosinophils
  Biopsy including artery, arteriole or venule, showing
    accumulations of eosinophils in extravascular areas

From Masi et al. [3]. With permission from John Wiley and Sons

8.3   Epidemiology

Among the three ANCA-associated vasculitides (EGPA, GPA and MPA), EGPA is the rarest with an annual incidence of 1–3 cases/million [4]. The median age at diagnosis is 50 years and there is a slight a male preponderance.

8.4   Etiology

The exact etiology of the condition is unknown, but the prominence of allergic features, the pronounced T-cell immunity with granuloma formation along with the increased globulin level, especially IgE and immune complex formation, all suggest an autoimmune process. It is thought that environmental and genetic factors (HLA-DRB4) may also play a role [5].

EGPA has been associated with the use of leukotriene therapies for asthma and anti-IgE monoclonal antibodies (omalizumab) [6]. In most instances, it is thought that the occurrence of EGPA reflects masking of previously undiagnosed EGPA in asthmatic patients taking glucocorticoids.

8.5   Clinical Manifestations

EGPA is believed to evolve through three clinical phases [2]:

1. Prodromal phase
   This phase may last for years and is characterized by asthma, with or without atopic features (e.g., allergic rhinitis, nasal polyposis).
2. Eosinophilic phase
   Peripheral blood eosinophilia and eosinophilic tissue infiltration often of the lung and gastrointestinal tract.
3. Vasculitic phase
   This is the most severe phase and may only become apparent several years after the initial or prodromal phase.
   Symptoms of malaise, lethargy, weight loss, and fevers are often experienced during the vasculitic phase of the disease.

8.5.1   Pulmonary

Asthma, usually late-onset (mean age 50 years), is a cardinal feature of the disease and seen in the majority of cases (>95 %). Corticosteroid use in asthma often masks the onset of vasculitis for many years. The asthma may worsen just before the onset of vasculitis, leading to hospital admissions.

8.5.2   Cutaneous

Skin involvement is seen in 40–70 % of patients and is one of the most common features of the vasculitic phase of EGPA (Fig. 8.1). It reflects the predilection for small vessels. Palpable purpura (50 %) commonly occurs on the lower

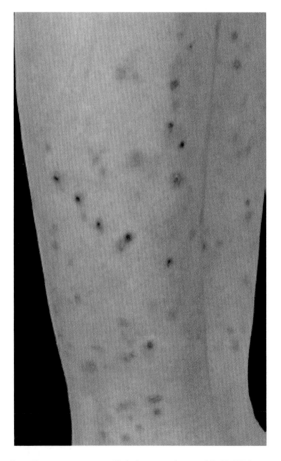

FIGURE 8.1 Cutaneous vasculitis in a patient with EGPA

extremities. Cutaneous or subcutaneous nodules (30 %) are the most distinctive skin lesions of EGPA, but not pathognomonic. These red or violaceous lesions occur primarily on the scalp and the limbs or hands and feet and are often bilateral and symmetrical.

8.5.3   Gastrointestinal

Gastrointestinal manifestations are the least common of EGPA complications (30 %), but very important to recognize.

Symptoms include abdominal pain, diarrhea (eosinophilic gastroenteritis or colitis), nausea, vomiting, and bleeding. Vasculitis and granulomata can be found throughout the gastrointestinal tract, but are more commonly seen in the small intestine or colon. Bowel ischemia can result from vasculitis of the small vessels and can be life-threatening if bowel perforation occurs. Involvement of the gastrointestinal tract is considered a factor of poor prognosis.

8.5.4   Neurological

The nervous system is a commonly involved system in EGPA (78 %). Peripheral neuropathy, often mononeuritis multiplex, and distal symmetrical or asymmetrical polyneuropathy have all been described. With treatment, mononeuritis multiplex can be reversed without sequelae. However, when sequelae are present, they are more sensory than motor.

Central nervous system involvement can present with confusion, seizures, and in severe cases, coma. Cranial nerve palsies are infrequent (Fig. 8.2), the most common cranial nerve lesion being ischemic optic neuropathy. Cerebral ischemic or hemorrhagic changes can be seen.

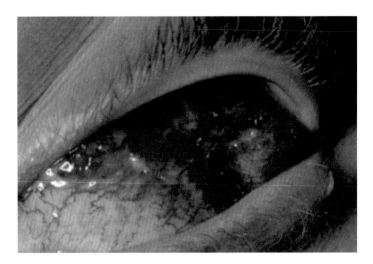

FIGURE 8.2 Ocular involvement with scleritis in patients with EGPA

8.5.5   Cardiac

Cardiac involvement is recognized as a poor prognostic factor and is found in approximately 44 % of patients and is the commonest cause of death in patients with EGPA. Pericarditis (acute or constrictive) due to eosinophilic pericardial disease can lead to cardiac tamponade. Cardiomyopathy (typically restrictive) due to endomyocardial fibrosis, myocardial infarction, arrhythmias (due to involvement of conductive tissue), and valvular disease (endocarditis) also occur.

8.5.6   Renal

Renal involvement is less common in EGPA (44 %), when compared to renal involvement in GPA or MPA, and in particular, renal failure is rare. Renal involvement has been demonstrated as one of the poor prognostic factors.

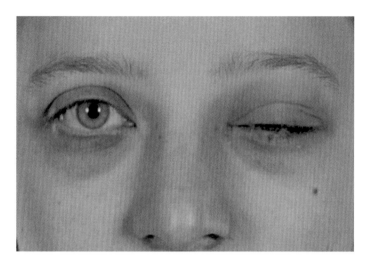

FIGURE 8.3   Ptosis in a patient with EGPA

8.5.7   ENT

Allergic rhinitis and sinus problems are very commonly seen in EGPA (70 %). Reported ENT manifestations include nasal obstruction, recurrent sinusitis, and polyp formation. Rarely, a chronic otitis picture, deafness, and skull base infiltration with eosinophilic granulomata may occur.

8.5.8   Ophthalmic

The eye can also be involved in EGPA and uveitis, episcleritis, conjunctival nodules, and retinal vasculitis have all been described. Eosinophilic infiltration may lead to exophthalmos, a rare complication of EGPA, which is often reversible (Fig. 8.3).

8.5.9   Musculoskeletal

Involvement of the muscles and joints is not uncommon in EGPA (57 %). This is often in the form of myalgias, migratory polyarthralgias, or frank arthritis. Joint deformity and radiographic erosions do not occur. Arthralgias often occur in the first few days or weeks with predominantly larger joint involvement. Myalgias are also frequent and usually improve quickly under treatment, but sometimes they can be so intense that they mimic polymyositis.

8.6   Laboratory Features

The FBC may show a normocytic, normochromic anemia. A differential white cell count typically shows an eosinophilia ($>1.5 \times 10^9$/L), which may be as high as 30×10^9/L. There is an acute phase response with raised inflammatory markers (ESR and CRP). Hypergammaglobulinemia/raised IgE occurs frequently.

8.6.1   Immunology

ANCA is positive in 50% of patients with active disease especially if there is renal involvement. Antimyeloperoxidase (MPO) antibodies (and/or pANCA) are most commonly detected.

8.6.2   Imaging

Fleeting, patchy pulmonary infiltrates, typically in the periphery of the lungs, occur in 50 % of patients with EGPA. Pleural effusions are seen in up to 10 % of patients and are a result of eosinophilic infiltration of the pleura or heart (congestive cardiac failure).

8.6.3   Pathology

Tissue and peripheral blood eosinophilia are the hallmarks of EGPA. The characteristic pathological features are necrotizing small vessel vasculitis, eosinophilic inflammation, and extra-vascular granulomata. The commonest renal histological abnormality is that of a pauci-immune focal segmental necro-tizing glomerulonephritis with crescent formation, similar to other ANCA-associated vasculitides.

8.7   Diagnosis

8.7.1   Differential Diagnosis

It is important to differentiate EGPA from the other vasculi-tides such as GPA, MPA, and polyarteritis nodosa. Also, it is important to distinguish it from other eosinophilic syn-dromes, e.g., idiopathic hypereosinophilic syndrome, chronic eosinophilic pneumonia, parasitic infections, allergic bron-chopulmonary aspergillosis, and drug reactions.

8.7.2   Assessment of Organ Involvement

Individual organ involvement should be assessed. Renal function tests are the most important, particularly urinalysis (see above). Urinalysis should be performed urgently in all patients, in whom systemic vasculitis is suspected, looking for proteinuria, hematuria, and red cell casts. Renal function may be assessed by creatinine clearance, 24-h urine protein excre-tion, or protein/creatinine ratios. In the presence of renal involvement, renal biopsy is important to assess the severity and extent of inflammation with the commonest finding being a focal segmental necrotizing glomerulonephritis, with few if any immune deposits. ECG and echocardiography are important tests to exclude any cardiac involvement, which can be life-threatening.

A chest X-ray may show transient and patchy opacities, hilar lymphadenopathy, septal thickening, or pleural effu-sions. Bronchoscopy can help demonstrate a predominant eosinophilic infiltrate in the bronchoalveolar lavage.

Other investigations are required, depending on clinical involvement. For example, nerve condition studies and neural biopsy can be helpful in the presence of neuropathy. Tissue biopsy of affected organs, e.g., skin, nerve, kidney, can help establish the diagnosis.

8.8   Assessment of Disease Activity

This can be performed using scoring systems such as The Birmingham Vasculitis Activity Score and Health Assessment Questionnaires (HAQ) for general health function. Involvement of target organs such as the heart, kidneys, and nerves (central and/or peripheral) usually signifies severe disease and has important prognostic value.

8.9   Treatment

Guidelines on the management of ANCA Associated Vasculitides have been recently published [7, 8]. Although the randomized controlled trials s included relatively few patients with EGPA, it is generally accepted that EGPA is treated using the same principles as GPA and MPA. The intensity of initial immunosuppression depends on the severity of organ involvement and size of vessels involved (Table 4.1; Fig. 4.1). Therefore, an important part of treatment planning involves assessment of organ involvement and its severity. Treatment may be divided into remission induction, maintenance, and long-term follow-up (see Chap. 4 for details).

8.9.1   Remission Induction

Remission induction is usually undertaken using a combination of corticosteroids and cyclophosphamide. Pulse intravenous cyclophosphamide is associated with similar responses to oral cyclophosphamide but fewer side effects, probably due to lower cumulative dosage. A number of regimens have been described; most use two-weekly intravenous cyclophosphamide, maximum 15 mg/kg (but reduce with renal impairment and age) for three consecutive infusions, thereafter reducing frequency to three weekly for between 3 and 6 months. Mesna may be used to reduce risk of bladder toxicity and intermittent oral septrin is advised for PCP prophylaxis. There is some data on the use of B cell depletion with Rituximab for remission induction as an alternative to pulse cyclophosphamide,

8.9.2   Maintenance

Once remission has been induced, oral Azathioprine or Methotrexate is the standard treatment, which need to be given for at least 18 months. In particularly severe disease, plasma exchange needs to be given in addition to the above remission induction.

8.10   Prognosis

Prognosis has significantly improved with the use of immuno-suppressant therapies, with reported 5-year survival rates in the range of 60–70 %. Overall prognosis at presentation is determined by the presence of neuropathy, renal involvement, and cardiac involvement. The five-factor score (see Fig. 10.2) predicts outcome. The presence of one prognostic factor gave a 5-year mortality of 12 %; two prognostic factors, a 5-year mortality of 26 %; and three or more prognostic factors, a 5-year mortality of 46 % [9].

Key Points
- EGPA is a rare, ANCA-associated vasculitis of small to medium vessels, characterized by the late-onset of asthma and eosinophilia.
- Corticosteroids form the basis of treatment, with the addition of cytotoxic agents such as cyclophosphamide when there is multiorgan involvement.

References

1. Jennette JC, Falk RJ, Bacon PA, et al. 2012 revised international chapel hill consensus conference nomenclature of vasculitides. Arthritis Rheum. 2013;65:1–11.
2. Lanham JG, Elkon KB, Pusey CD, Hughes GR. Systemic vasculitis with asthma and eosinophilia: a clinical approach to the Churg-Strauss syndrome. Medicine. 1984;63:65–81.
3. Masi AT, Hunder GG, Lie JT, et al. The American College of Rheumatology 1990 criteria for the classification of Churg-Strauss syndrome (allergic granulomatosis angiitis). Arthritis Rheum. 1990;33:1094–100.
4. Watts RA, Scott DGI. Epidemiology of vasculitis. In: Ball GV, Bridges L, editors. Vasculitis. 3rd ed. Oxford: Oxford University Press; 2014. p. 7–28.
5. Wieczorek S, Hellmich B, Arning L, et al. Functionally relevant variations of the interleukin-10 gene associated with antineutrophil cytoplasmic antibody-negative Churg-Strauss syndrome, but not with Wegener's granulomatosis. Arthritis Rheum. 2008; 58:1839.
6. Wechsler M, Wong D, Miller MK, Lawrence-Miyasaki L. Churg Strauss syndrome in patients treated with omalizumab. Chest. 2009;136:507–18.
7. Ntatsaki E, Carruthers D, Chakravarty K, D'Cruz D, Harper L, Jayne DRW, Luqmani RA, Venning M, Mooney J, Mills J, Watts RA. BSR and BHPR guidelines for the management of adults with ANCA associated vasculitis. Rheumatology. 2014;53(1): 145–528.
8. Mukhtyar C, Guillevin L, Cid M, et al. EULAR recommendations for the management of primary small and medium vessel vasculitis. Ann Rheum Dis. 2009;68:310–7.
9. Guillevin L, Lhote F, Gavraud M, et al. Prognostic factors in polyarteritis nodosa and Churg-Strauss syndrome. A prospective study in 342 patients. Medicine (Baltimore). 1996;75:17–28.

Chapter 9
Microscopic Polyangiitis

9.1 Introduction

Microscopic polyangiitis (MPA) is a medium, small-vessel vasculitis characterized by pauci immune glomerulonephritis, pulmonary involvement, and the presence of ANCA. It was first described by Davson in 1948 and called microscopic polyarteritis, it was more widely recognized following the discovery of the association with ANCA.

9.2 Definition and Classification

The Chapel Hill Consensus conference in 2012 defined MPA in the ANCA associated group as "Necrotizing vasculitis, with few or no immune deposits, predominantly affecting small vessels (i.e. capillaries, venules, or arterioles). Necrotizing arteritis involving small and medium-sized arteries may be present. Necrotizing glomerulonephritis is very common. Pulmonary capillaritis often occurs. Granulomatous inflammation is absent." [1] The ACR did not consider MPA in their 1990 classification scheme. There are no validated diagnostic criteria.

R.A. Watts et al., *Vasculitis in Clinical Practice*,
DOI 10.1007/978-3-319-14871-7_9,
© Springer International Publishing AG, Cham 2015

9.3   Epidemiology

The annual incidence of MPA in the UK is approximately 5/million with a prevalence of approximately 100/million. The peak age of onset is 65–75 years and it is more common in men than women. It is very rare in childhood. There is evidence for variation in incidence between populations. In Europe, MPA appears to be more common than GPA in the South, while the reverse is true in the North of Europe [2]. In Japan, MPA is the predominant form of ANCA-associated vasculitis.

9.4   Etiology

The etiology of MPA is unknown but like most autoimmune conditions is believed to result from the interaction of trigger factors with a genetically predisposed host. ANCA in animals have been shown to be pathogenic. ANCA can activate TNF-alpha primed neutrophils, inducing production of reactive oxygen species and release of proteolytic enzymes including ANCA-target antigens.

9.5   Clinical Features

9.5.1   Systemic

Many patients describe a prodromal systemic illness with fever (45 %), weight loss (35–60 %), myalgia (40 %), and arthralgia (30–60 %). This may precede the onset of fulminant disease by up to 2 years [3, 4].

9.5.2   Renal

Renal involvement is seen in most patients (up to 90 %) with MPA and is the most common organ involved. An active urinary sediment may be present, with red cells and red cell casts which are characteristic of glomerular involvement.

Rapidly progressive glomerulonephritis is common leading to acute or subacute renal failure and up to 20 % require dialysis. Proteinuria is common and, rarely, a nephrotic syndrome may develop. The prognosis is determined by the extent of renal involvement.

9.5.3   Pulmonary

Pulmonary involvement is common in MPA and may vary clinically from mild dyspnoea to life-threatening massive pulmonary hemorrhage. Pulmonary hemorrhage occurs in up to 30 % of patients with MPA and is associated with a worse prognosis. Pulmonary fibrosis may develop as a consequence of pulmonary hemorrhage. Patients present with dyspnoea and hemoptysis; the chest radiograph shows patchy alveolar shadowing (Figs. 9.1 and 9.2). Nodular or cavitating lesions on

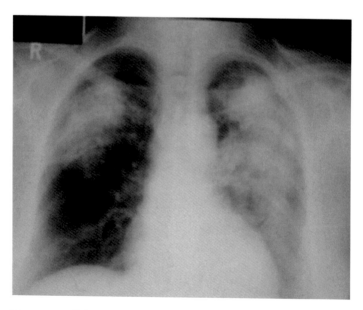

FIGURE 9.1   CXR showing pulmonary hemorrhage in a patient with microscopic polyangiitis (MPA)

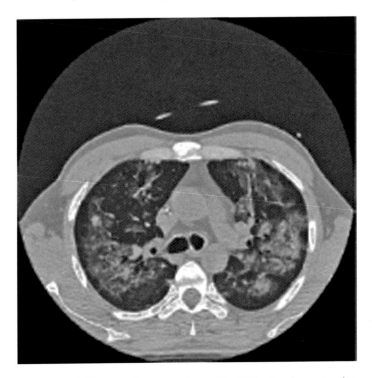

FIGURE 9.2 CT thorax from a patient with MPA showing extensive pulmonary hemorrhage

a chest radiograph suggest granulomatous lesions more typical of GPA. Pulmonary function tests undertaken during active pulmonary hemorrhage show a raised K_{CO}, and blood- or hemosiderinladen macrophages are found at bronchoalveolar lavage.

9.5.4   Cutaneous

Skin involvement is frequent (36 % at diagnosis, 25–60 % overall), typically a purpuric rash. Nailbed infarcts, splinter hemorrhages, livedo, infarction, or ulceration can occur.

9.5.5   Neurological

Neuropathy occurs in up to 30 % of patients. Peripheral neuropathy is more common than mononeuritis multiplex affecting either peripheral or cranial nerves. Cerebral vasculitis is rare but may manifest with cerebral hemorrhage infarction seizures or headache.

9.5.6   Cardiac

Cardiac involvement is rare (3 %) but pericarditis and cardiac failure have been reported. This is in contrast to CSS, which is also associated with MPO-ANCA, in which cardiac disease is one of the predominant features (occurring in 26 %).

9.5.7   Gastrointestinal

Abdominal pain, diarrhea, and gastrointestinal bleeding occur in 30 % but are less common than in PAN.

9.5.8   Otorhinolaryngeal

Mild symptoms of rhinitis, epistaxis, and sinusitis are compatible with a diagnosis of MPA but severe destructive disease, infiltrative, or granulomatous disease is not seen and its occurrence is highly suggestive of GPA.

9.5.9   Ocular

Florid uveitis, retinal vasculitis, optic neuropathy, and orbital granulomata occur more commonly in GPA rather than MPA, where a mild episcleritis may occur in 20 %.

9.5.10   Venous Thromboembolism

Venous thomboembolism is a common occurrence in MPA, occurring in around 7.6 % of patients within a median 5.8 months from diagnosis.

9.6   Laboratory Features

MPA is a systemic inflammatory illness and therefore there is often a marked acute phase response with a nonspecific elevation of ESR and CRP, a mild normochromic normocytic anemia, thrombocytosis and low serum albumin. Eosinophilia is not characteristic of MPA and if present is suggestive of EGPA.

9.6.1   Immunology

Perinuclear ANCA with an anti-MPO specificity is characteristically found [5]. A few patients are cANCA positive with PR3 specificity. ANA and RF may be present but are typically negative. Complement levels are normal. Anti-GBM antibodies are not present.

9.6.2   Pathology

The characteristic distinguishing features of MPA pathology are found in the kidney and lung. The typical renal lesion is a focal and segmental glomerulonephritis with fibrinoid necrosis of the glomerular capillary wall leading to crescent formation (Fig. 9.3). There is little or no endocapillary proliferation. Immunofluorescence shows few or absent immune deposits (pauci-immune). These features are similar to those seen in Wegener's granulomatosis and idiopathic rapidly progressive crescentic glomerulonephritis, although those in MPA tend to show a more chronic pattern with more interstitial

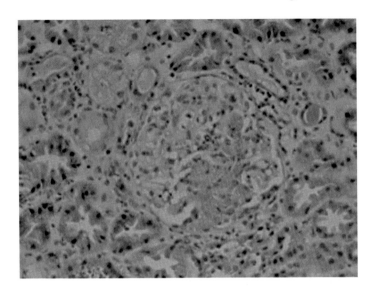

FIGURE 9.3 Renal biopsy from a patient with MPA, showing segmental glomerular necrosis, fibrin deposition, and neutrophil polymorph infiltration

fibrosis, tubular atrophy, and glomerulosclerosis. Capillaritis is the underlying pathological feature in the lung, and very infrequently, immune deposits are found. Interstitial fibrosis after recurrent episodes of alveolar hemorrhage is now well recognized, especially in MPO-ANCA positive patients [6]. In the skin there is a pauci-immune necrotizing leukocytoclastic vasculitis.

9.7   Diagnosis

9.7.1   Differential Diagnosis

There is an overlap between MPA and GPA, and this can make the differential diagnosis difficult in the early stages. This is not critical as the treatment approach is almost identical. Anti-GBM disease (Goodpasture's syndrome) can be distinguished by the presence of antiglomerular basement membrane antibodies. Other causes of a systemic illness such as infection (endocarditis), mimics of vasculitis (cholesterol embolism, atrial myxoma, calciphylaxis, malignancy) need to be excluded.

9.7.2   Assessment of Organ Involvement

Individual organ involvement should be assessed. In patients suspected of a systemic vasculitis, urinalysis (looking for proteinuria, hematuria, red cell casts) should be performed urgently. Renal function should be assessed by creatinine clearance, quantification of protein leak, if present using urine protein/creatinine ratio. A chest radiograph should be performed in all patients looking for the evidence of pulmonary hemorrhage, infection, or nodules. Other organ involvement should be assessed as appropriate, for example nerve conduction studies looking for evidence of neuropathy.

9.8   Assessment of Disease Activity

Several scoring systems have been developed to objectively determine disease extent and activity; these include the Disease Extent Index (DEI) and the Birmingham Vasculitis Activity Score (BVAS) [7]. The BVAS has been validated. Damage as a consequence of vasculitis can be assessed using the vasculitis damage index (VDI). Quality of life can be assessed using the SF-36.

The utility of serial determinations of ANCA to predict relapse, and hence changes in therapy has been controversial [8]. Overall low predictive values for relapse were found, and so it is not justified to escalate immunosuppressive therapy solely on the basis of an increase in ANCA level, as determined by PR3/MPO ELISA. An increase should be taken as a warning and the patient observed more closely. The aim of the therapy is to induce and maintain remission with a minimum tissue damage due to either disease activity or therapy.

9.9   Treatment

Guidelines on the management of MPA have been recently published [9, 10]. The intensity of initial immunosuppression depends on the severity of organ involvement and size of vessels involved (Table 4.1; Fig. 4.1). Therefore an important part of treatment planning involves assessment of organ involvement and its severity. Treatment may be divided into remission induction, maintenance, and long-term follow-up (see Chap. 4 for details).

9.9.1   Remission Induction

Remission induction is usually undertaken using a combination of corticosteroids and cyclophosphamide. Pulse intravenous cyclophosphamide is associated with similar responses to oral cyclophosphamide but fewer side-effects, probably due to lower cumulative dosage. A number of regimens have been described; most use two-weekly intravenous cyclophosphamide, maximum 15 mg/kg (but reduce with renal impairment and age) for three consecutive infusions, thereafter reducing frequency to three weekly for between 3 and 6 months. Mesna may be used to reduce risk of bladder toxicity and intermittent oral septrin is advised for PCP prophylaxis. B cell depletion with Rituximab is an alternative treatment for remission induction [11, 12] and is used when there are concerns for fertility or other contraindications to the use of cyclophosphamide. Rituximab is also often used for relapsing disease as there is evidence that the long term toxicity of cyclophosphamide is closely related to the cumulative doe – the risk being particularly high at cumulative doses over 15 g.

The frequency of severe renal failure is greater in MPA than in GPA or EGPA and for these patients plasma exchange should be considered (see Fig. 4.1). A recent RCT compared plasma exchange and pulsed methylprednisolone as an adjunctive therapy in biopsy-proven AAV with acute renal failure (creatinine >500 μmol/L). Renal outcome was better in the plasma exchange-treated group when expressed as either dialysis independence in surviving patients or overall rate of dialysis-free survival. Death rates were similar in both groups. These results were maintained at 1-year follow-up [13].

9.9.2   Maintenance

Once remission has been induced, oral azathioprine or methotrexate is the standard treatment which needs to be given for at least 18 months. In particularly severe disease, plasma exchange needs to be given in addition to the above remission induction therapy.

When Rituximab is used for remission induction or for relapse, there may not be any requirement for additional immunosuppression with these drugs.

9.10   Prognosis

The 1-year survival in patients with a new diagnosis of MPA using the treatment approach described above is 84 %, with a 5-year survival of 45 % [4]. The overall outcome for MPA is generally worse than for either GPA or EGPA, which reflects the-older age and worse renal function at presentation. Survival is lower in patients with initially raised creatinine and in those with end-stage renal disease, at 64 % at 1 year and 53 % at 5 years. Pulmonary hemorrhage is the worst predictor of poor outcome with an eightfold relative risk of death [14]. Relapse is higher in patients with pANCA/MPO compared with cANCA/PR3 but ANCA specificity in most studies does not affect early survival or renal outcome.

The five factor score (see Fig. 10.2) predicts outcome. The presence of one prognostic factor gave a 5-year mortality of 12 %; two prognostic factors, a 5-year mortality of 26 %; and three or more prognostic factors, a 5-year mortality of 46 % [15].

Key Points
- MPA is a medium small vessel vasculitis characterized by a pulmonary renal syndrome.
- pANCA/MPO is typically present in serum.
- Treatment is with cyclophosphamide and glucocorticoids to induce remission.

References

1. Jennette JC, Falk RJ, Bacon PA, et al. 2012 Revised international Chapel Hill Consensus Conference nomenclature of vasculitides. Arthritis Rheum. 2013;65:1–11.
2. Watts RA, Scott DGI. Epidemiology of vasculitis. In: Ball GV, Fessler BJ, Bridges SL, editors. Oxford textbook of vasculitis. 3rd ed. Oxford: Oxford University Press; 2014. p. 7–25.
3. Savage CO, Winearls CG, Evans DJ, Rees AJ. Microscopic polyarteritis: presentation, pathology and prognosis. Q J Med. 1985;56:467–83.
4. Lane SE, Watts RA, Scott DGI. Primary systemic vasculitis: clinical features and mortality. Q J Med. 2005;98:97–112.
5. Choi HK, Liu S, Merkel PA, Colditz GA, Niles JL. Diagnostic performance of antineutrophil cytoplasmic antibody tests for idiopathic vasculitides: metaanalysis with a focus on antimyeloperoxidase antibodies. J Rheumatol. 2001;28:1584–90.
6. Homma S, Matsushita H, Nakata K. Pulmonary fibrosis in myeloperoxidase antineutrophil cytoplasmic antibody-associated vasculitides. Respirology. 2004;9:190–6.
7. Luqmani RA. Assessment of disease activity and damage. In: Ball GV, Fessler BJ, Bridges SL, editors. Oxford textbook of vasculitis. 3rd ed. Oxford: Oxford University Press; 2014. p. 299–305.
8. Birck R, Schmitt W, Kaelsch IA, van Der Woude FJ. Serial ANCA determinations *for monitoring* disease activity in patients with ANCA-associated vasculitis: systematic review. Am J Kidney Dis. 2006;47:15–23.
9. Ntatsaki E, Carruthers D, Chakravarty K, et al. BSR/BHPR guideline for the management of adults with ANCA-associated vasculitis. Rheumatology. 2014. doi:10.1093/rheumatology/ket445.

10. Mukhtyar C, Guillevin L, Cid M, et al. EULAR recommenda-
    tions for the management of primary small and medium vessel
    vasculitis. Ann Rheum Dis. 2009;68:310–7.
11. Jones RB, Tervaert JW, Hauser T, et al. Rituximab versus cyclo-
    phosphamide in ANCA-associated renal vasculitis. N Engl J
    Med. 2010;363:211–20.
12. Stone JH, Merkel PA, Spiera R, et al. Rituximab versus cyclo-
    phosphamide for ANCA-associated vasculitis. N Engl J Med.
    2010;363:221–32.
13. Jayne DR, Gaskin G, Rasmussen N, et al. Randomised trial of
    plasma exchange and high-dosage methylprednisolone as
    adjunctive therapy for severe renal vasculitis. J Am Soc Nephrol.
    2007;18:2180–8.
14. Hogan SL, Nachman PH, Wilkman AS, Jennette JC, Falk
    RJ. Prognostic markers in patients with antineutrophil cytoplas-
    mic autoantibody-associated microscopic polyangiitis and glo-
    merulonephritis. J Am Soc Nephrol. 1996;7:23–32.
15. Guillevin L, Lhote F, Gavraud M, et al. Prognostic factors in
    polyarteritis nodosa and Churg-Strauss syndrome. A prospective
    study in 342 patients. Medicine (Baltimore). 1996;75:17–28.

Chapter 10
Polyarteritis Nodosa

10.1 Introduction

Polyarteritis nodosa (PAN) is a rare medium vessel vasculitis that is often associated with Hepatitis B Virus (HBV-PAN) infection. It was first described by Kussmaul and Meier in 1866, in a patient with palpable cutaneous nodules.

10.2 Definition and Classification

The Chapel Hill Consensus Conference in 1994 defined cPAN as "Necrotizing inflammation of medium-sized or small arteries without glomerulonephritis or vasculitis in arterioles, capillaries, or venules; and not associated with ANCA" [1]. The ACR in 1990 developed classification criteria that are widely used in clinical trials (Table 10.1) [2]. The criteria have a sensitivity of 82.2 % and specificity of 86.6 %. There are no validated diagnostic criteria.

10.3 Epidemiology

PAN as defined by the CHCC is very rare with an annual incidence of <1/million [3]. In areas endemic for HBV, incidence rates of up to 77/million have been recorded. PAN

R.A. Watts et al., *Vasculitis in Clinical Practice*,
DOI 10.1007/978-3-319-14871-7_10,
© Springer International Publishing AG, Cham 2015

TABLE 10.1 ACR (1990) classification criteria for PAN

Weight loss

  Loss of 4 kg or more of body weight since the illness began, not due to dieting or other factors

Livedo reticularis

  Mottled reticular pattern over the skin of portions of the extremities or torso

Testicular pain or tenderness

  Pain or tenderness of the testicles, not due to infection, trauma, or other causes

Myalgias, weakness, or leg tenderness

  Diffuse myalgias (excluding shoulder or hip girdle) or weakness of muscles or tenderness of leg muscles

Mononeuropathy or polyneuropathy

  Development of mononeuropathy, multiple mononeuropathies, or polyneuropathy

Diastolic BP >90 mmHg

  Development of hypertension with diastolic BP >90 mmHg

Elevated blood urea or creatinine

  Elevated BUN >40 mg/dL or creatinine 1.5 mg/dL, not due to dehydration or obstruction

Hepatitis B virus (HBV)

  Presence of hepatitis B surface antigen or antibody in serum

Arteriographic abnormality

  Arteriogram showing aneurysms or occlusion of the visceral arteries, not due to arteriosclerosis, fibromuscular dysplasia, or other noninflammatory causes

Table 10.1 (continued)

Biopsy of small or medium vessel
Histological changes showing the presence of sized artery containing PMN granulocytes or granulocytes and mononuclear leucocytes in the artery wall

Note for purposes of classification a patient shall be said to have PAN if at least three of these ten criteria are present (Lightfoot et al. [2]) With permission from John Wiley and Sons

occurs at all ages and is more common in men. The incidence of HBV-PAN has been falling due to increased vaccination against HBV and screening of blood products for HBV infection. The most common cause now is drug abuse.

10.4   Etiology

The etiology of PAN is unknown. There is clear evidence that in HBV the formation of immune complexes containing HBsAg is the triggering factor. ANCA and other autoantibodies are not found in PAN suggesting that it is not a classical autoimmune disease. No clear HLA associations have been established.

10.5   Clinical Features

The spectrum of disease severity is broad ranging from mild, limited disease to progressive disease, which may be fatal. Virtually any organ may eventually be affected. The clinical features of PAN and HBV-PAN are similar [4, 5].

10.5.1   Systemic

Typically, the patient experiences constitutional features of fever, malaise, weight loss, and diffuse aching, along with manifestations of multisystem involvement such as peripheral neuropathy and an asymmetric polyarthritis. Visceral involvement, such as the kidney or gut, may present coincidentally with these features or may appear later.

10.5.2   Cutaneous

Cutaneous lesions include infarctions, ulcerations, livedo reticularis, subcutaneous nodules, and ischemic changes of the distal digits (Fig. 10.1) and occur in 25–60 % of patients.

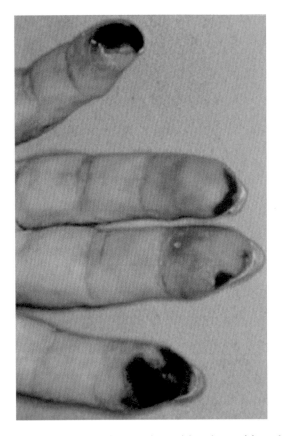

Figure 10.1 Digital ischemia in patient with polyarteritis nodosa

10.5.3   Musculoskeletal

Arthralgia or arthritis is present in as many as 50 % of patients. A polymyalgic syndrome may occur at presentation. An asymmetric, episodic, nondeforming polyarthritis involving the larger joints of the lower extremity may occur in up to 20 % of cases, most commonly early in the disease.

10.5.4   Neurological

Peripheral neuropathy may occur in up to 70 % of cPAN and may be the initial manifestation. The neuropathy affects the lower extremities somewhat more often than the upper extremities. The onset is often very acute, with pain and paresthesias radiating in the distribution of a peripheral nerve, followed in hours by a motor deficit of the same peripheral nerve. This may progress asymmetrically to involve other peripheral nerves and produce a mononeuritis multiplex or a multiple mononeuropathy. With additional nerve damage, the final result may be a symmetric polyneuropathy involving all sensory modalities and motor functions. CNS involvement is much less common and includes headache, seizures, cranial nerve dysfunction, cerebral hemorrhage, and stroke.

10.5.5   Renal

PAN is usually characterized by vascular nephropathy, without glomerulonephritis in about 35 % of patients. Multiple renal infarcts, the consequence of vascular nephropathy, produce renal failure. Renal angiography will frequently show several aneurysms and infarcts. Ureteral stenosis and perinephric hematomas (microaneurysm rupture) can occur. Hypertension develops as a result of renal artery or, less commonly, renal parenchymal involvement. Hypertension, usually mild, occurs in 21–33 % of patients and is particularly associated with hepatitis B infection.

10.5.6   Gastrointestinal

Abdominal pain occurs in up to 70 % of patients. Features of gastrointestinal involvement include abdominal pain, diarrhea, gut hemorrhage, and abnormal liver enzyme tests. Liver involvement is not common clinically, except if associated with hepatitis B infection. Gastrointestinal involvement is among the most serious features of PAN and is associated with a poor prognosis. Abdominal pain due to vasculitis may be the first manifestation of vasculitis and presents a particular challenge.

10.5.7   Cardiac

Cardiac involvement is common pathologically, but is recognized less often clinically. Myocardial infarction, when it occurs, is usually silent and is due to coronary arteritis. Cardiomegaly occurs in about 20 % of patients. Congestive heart failure develops as a result of coronary insufficiency or severe hypertension (or both). Cardiomyopathy is predictive of increased mortality. Endocarditis is not observed in PAN and its occurrence should alert the clinician to an alternative diagnosis.

10.5.8   Orchitis

Testicular involvement is manifested by pain, but clinical involvement indicated by swelling or induration occurs only in a small percentage of patients. Orchitis is one of the most characteristic features of PAN and is more common in polyarteritis complicated by gastrointestinal involvement and, in particular, vasculitis associated with hepatitis B. It is rarely the first manifestation of the disease, usually unilateral, and is caused by ischemia of the testicular artery.

10.5.9   Other

Pulmonary involvement is so uncommon in PAN that other causes should be sought, especially infection. Diffuse involvement of skeletal muscle arteries may cause ischemic pain and intermittent claudication. Myalgias occur in about 50 % of cases of polyarteritis, but generalized myopathy and increased creatine kinase concentrations are unusual. Venous thromboembolism is less common than in MPA occurring in 2.8 % of patients.

10.6   Laboratory Features

PAN is a systemic inflammatory illness, and therefore, there is often a marked acute phase response with a nonspecific elevation of ESR and CRP, a mild normochromic normocytic anemia, thrombocytosis, and low serum albumin.

10.6.1   Immunology

PAN with or without HBV infection is not associated with ANCA. Rheumatoid factor, ANA, cryoglobulins, and anticardiolipin antibodies are negative or normal.

10.6.2   Viral Serology

Evidence of viral infection should be sort, especially HBV and HCV.

10.6.3   Imaging

Contrast angiography may be the diagnostic procedure of choice in hepatitis B-associated polyarteritis. The typical angiographic appearance includes long segments of smooth arterial stenosis alternating with areas of normal or dilated artery, smooth tapered occlusions, thrombosis, and the lack of significant atherosclerosis. The dilated segments include saccular and fusiform aneurysms, which strongly suggest classic polyarteritis nodosa (Fig. 10.2). The most frequently involved vessels are the renal, hepatic, and mesenteric vessels. When

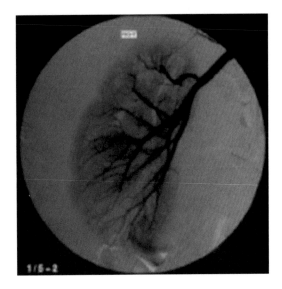

FIGURE 10.2 Angiogram from a patient with polyarteritis nodosa showing microaneurysms

angiography is performed, it is important that all intraabdominal vessels are studied, including the coeliac axis, mesenteric, renal, and hepatic arteries. The angiographic appearances may regress after treatment. The role of MRA is not established.

10.6.4   Pathology

The pathology of polyarteritis consists of focal, necrotizing inflammatory lesions, which extend through the wall of small and medium-sized arteries. The inflammation is characterized by fibrinoid necrosis and pleomorphic cellular infiltration, with predominantly macrophages and lymphocytes and variable numbers of neutrophils and eosinophils (Fig. 10.3). A significant eosinophilic infiltrate favors the diagnosis of EGPA. The normal architecture of the vessel wall, including the elastic lamina, is disrupted. There may be

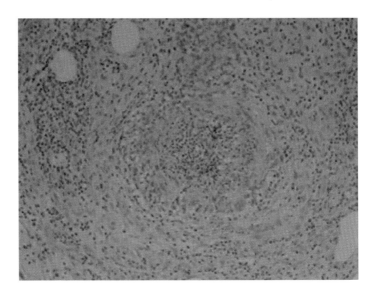

FIGURE. 10.3 Biopsy from a patient with polyarteritis nodosa showing a small subcutaneous artery with necrotizing inflammation of its wall and obliteration of its lumen by neutrophil polymorphs

thrombosis or aneurysmal dilation at the site of the lesion. Healed areas of arteritis show proliferation of fibrous tissue and endothelial cells, which may lead to vessel occlusion. Lesions at all stages of progression and healing may be seen pathologically if sufficient tissue is available for study. The focal nature of the inflammation increases the risk of a false-negative biopsy when the tissue sample is small. The finding of a perivascular inflammation or intimal proliferation without fibrinoid necrosis of the arterial wall suggests, but does not confirm, the diagnosis of polyarteritis. In autopsy studies of patients with classic polyarteritis nodosa, inflammation in the arcuate and interlobar arteries and arterioles of the kidney is frequently found, along with the evidence of infarction.

Muscle biopsy is positive in around 50 % of patients with PAN who have muscle pain or claudication. The yield on muscle biopsy is lower in asymptomatic cases.

10.7   Diagnosis

10.7.1   Differential Diagnosis

The differential diagnosis is from other types of vasculitis, infection, or malignancy. The diagnosis is often made on either tissue biopsy or angiography. Angiographic features including aneurysms, though typical of PAN, can occur in other conditions such as myxoma and bacterial endocarditis.

10.7.2   Assessment of Organ Involvement

Individual organ involvement should be assessed with biopsy as appropriate.

10.8   Assessment of Disease Activity

Several scoring systems have been developed to objectively determine disease extent and activity; these include the Disease Extent Index (DEI) and the Birmingham Vasculitis Activity Score (BVAS) [6]. The BVAS has been validated. Damage as a consequence of vasculitis can be assessed using the vasculitis damage index (VDI) [7]. Quality of life can be assessed using the SF-36.

10.9   Treatment

10.9.1   Non-HBV-PAN

A number of randomized controlled trials have been performed, but they include patients with CSS and precede the introduction of the CHCC definitions for PAN and MPA.

An analysis of four prospective trials including patients with PAN carried out between 1980 and 1993 [8] suggested

TABLE 10.2 Five-factor score (FFS) for prognosis of polyarteritis nodosa

Proteinuria >1 g/24 h
Serum creatinine >140 µmol/L
Gastrointestinal involvement
Cardiomyopathy
CNS involvement

From Guillevin et al. [10]
Score 1 point for each of these items present

that cyclophosphamide should be used in patients with severe disease as assessed using the 5 factor score (Table 10.2).

10.9.2   Virus-Associated PAN

The best treatment strategy for patients with systemic vasculitis associated with viral infection should take into account the etiology of the disease and be adapted to pathogenesis [5]. The combination of plasma exchange (PE) and anti-viral treatment is effective in HBV-PAN. Although cyclophosphamide and steroids in the doses outlined above are also effective, they allow the virus to persist which increases the chance of chronic hepatitis and/or liver cirrhosis developing and is therefore not the preferred first regimen. Antiviral drugs which have been used with benefit include vidarabine, interferon-α, and lamivudine [5], the latter giving the best results. Lamivudine (100 mg/day) is used with PE after a few days of steroids (the dose should be reduced in patients with renal impairment) and this regime is associated with 90 % recovery and 60 % seroconversion to anti-HBe. PE is started four times per week for 3 weeks, three times per week for 2–3 weeks, and then progressive lengthening between sessions. The response clinically can be very rapid, with recovery within 3 weeks. PE should be stopped with the detection of antihepatitis B antibodies (to avoid their clearance as well). There is little experience of TNF-α blockade or B-cell depletion in PAN.

10.10   Prognosis

The natural history of untreated PAN is of a rapidly progressive, usually fatal disease. Treated PAN can be considered to be a monophasic self-limiting disease that tends not to recur once remission is induced. Survival rates are 76–89 % for PAN (5) and 64–70 % for HBV-PAN [5]. During a mean follow up of 68.3 months 28 % of non-HBV PAN relapsed compared with 11 % of HBV PAN and 20 % of non-PAN died compared with 34 % of HBV PAN [9].

The Five-Factor Score (FFS) at presentation is a useful guide to prognosis (Table 10.2) [10]. A FFS of >2 in PAN is associated with a greatly increased mortality, which is improved by the use of CYC. In non-HBV cases, the major cause of death in HBV-PAN is gastrointestinal tract involvement. The majority of deaths in PAN are due to active vasculitis. Predictors of mortality are age at onset, together with CNS and cardiac involvement.

Key Points
- Rare medium vessel necrotizing vasculitis
- Typically ANCA negative in distinction to MPA
- Often associated with HBV infection
- Treatment for HBV-PAN is with antiviral therapy and PE

References

1. Jennette JC, Falk RJ, Bacon PA, et al. 2012 revised international Chapel Hill Consensus Conference nomenclature of vasculitides. Arthritis Rheum. 2013;65:1–11.
2. Lightfoot Jr RW, Michel BA, Bloch DA, et al. The American College of Rheumatology 1990 criteria for the classification of polyarteritis nodosa. Arthritis Rheum. 1990;33:1088–93.
3. Watts RA, Scott DGI. Epidemiology of vasculitis. In: Ball GV, Fessler BJ, Bridges SL, editors. Oxford textbook of vasculitis. 3rd ed. Oxford: Oxford University Press; 2014. p. 7–25.

4. Guillevin L, Terrier B. Polyarteritis nodosa. In: Ball GV, Fessler BJ, Bridges SL, editors. Oxford textbook of vasculitis. 3rd ed. Oxford: Oxford University Press; 2014. p. 331–50.

5. Guillevin L, Mahr A, Callard P, et al. Hepatitis B virus associated polyarteritis nodosa: clinical characteristics, outcome and impact of treatment in 115 patients. Medicine (Baltimore). 2005;84:313–22.

6. Luqmani RA. Assessment of disease activity and damage. In: Ball GV, Fessler BJ, Bridges SL, editors. Oxford textbook of vasculitis. 3rd ed. Oxford: Oxford University Press; 2014. p. 299–305.

7. Exley AR, Bacon PA, Luqmani RA, et al. Development and initial validation of the Vasculitis Damage Index for the standardized clinical assessment of damage in the systemic vasculitides. Arthritis Rheum. 1997;40:371–80.

8. Gayraud M, Guillevin L, Toumelin PL, et al. Long-term follow up of polyarteritis nodosa, microscopic polyangiitis and Churg Strauss syndrome: analysis of 4 prospective trials including 278 patients. Arthritis Rheum. 2001;44:668–77.

9. Pagnoux C, Seror R, Henegar C, et al. Clinical features and outcomes in 348 patients with polyarteritis nodosa: a systematic retrospective study of patients diagnosed between 1963 and 2005 and entered into the French Vasculitis Study group database. Arthritis Rheum. 2010;62:616–26.

10. Guillevin L, Pagnoux C, Seror R, et al. The five factor score revisited: assessment of prognosis systemic necrotizing vasculitides based on the French Vasculitis Study Group (FVSG) cohort. Medicine (Baltimore). 2011;90:19–27.

Chapter 11
Kawasaki Disease

11.1 Introduction

Kawasaki disease was first recognized in 1967 as an acute febrile mucocutaneous syndrome, but coronary arterial involvement was not recognized until 1973 [1]. In a study of 20 patients who had coronary angiography following abatement of their initial febrile illness, 12 of the 20 were found to have abnormal coronary angiograms with evidence of coronary aneurysms. Until this time, Kawasaki disease was thought to be a benign illness.

11.2 Definition and Classification

The Chapel Hill consensus conference defined Kawasaki disease as "Arteritis associated with the mucocutaneous lymph node syndrome and predominantly affecting medium and small arteries. Coronary arteries are often involved. Aorta and large arteries may be involved. Usually occurs in infants and young children" [2].

The original diagnostic criteria for KD were developed by the Japanese in 1984. These have been revised by the European League against Rheumatism and the Paediatric Rheumatology European Society (Table 11.1) [3].

R.A. Watts et al., *Vasculitis in Clinical Practice*,
DOI 10.1007/978-3-319-14871-7_11,
© Springer International Publishing AG, Cham 2015

TABLE 11.1 EULAR/PReS classification criteria for Kawasaki disease

Fever persisting for at least 5 days (mandatory criterion) plus any four of the following features:
Changes in peripheral extremities or perineal area
Polymorphous exanthema
Bilateral conjunctival injection
Changes of lips and oral cavity: injection of oral and phalangeal mucosa
Cervical lymphadenopathy

From Ozen et al. [3], with permission from BMJ Publishing Group Ltd

11.3   Epidemiology

Kawasaki disease is predominantly a disease affecting children less than 4 years of age. It is more prevalent in the Japanese and other Far Eastern ethnic populations than in the Caucasian population, but occurs worldwide. The annual incidence in Japan is 240/100,000 children under 5 years of age [4]. In England the incidence is about 14.6/100,000 children less than 5 years of age from the Indian subcontinent and 4.6/100,000 in Caucasian White [5]. The annual incidence appears to be rising in various parts of the world as reported from Canada [6], India [7] and Japan [4]. There seems to be a predilection for the boys with a ratio of 1.5:1. There is a seasonal variation in the extra-tropical regions with highest incidence from January to March in the northern hemisphere [8].

11.4   Etiology

The etiology of KD is unknown. In Japan epidemics have been documented suggesting an infectious etiology probably respiratory, but no specific viral or bacterial infection has so far been identified. There are similarities between KD and toxic shock syndrome which has led to the suggestion that superantigen activation is responsible for KD.

11.5   Clinical Features

Children with Kawasaki disease are usually less than 5 years of age. They have a persistent fever and are extremely irritable.

It is important to recognize that the clinical features can appear sequentially and there will be children who do not develop all the features of the disease. There are no ethnic variations in the clinical presentation.

11.5.1   Mucosal

Mucosal inflammation can involve the lips and the oral cavity. Labial involvement can vary from mild erythema to fissuring, peeling, and bleeding. The glossitis of Kawasaki disease has been likened to a strawberry tongue. Cervical lymphadenopathy is usually unilateral. The glands do not suppurate, are not tender, and classically enlarge to >1.5 cm in diameter.

11.5.2   Cutaneous

An erythematous rash of the palms and soles appears within 5 days of the fever (Fig. 11.1). The rash desquamates during the convalescent stage. Typically, patients with Kawasaki disease develop erythema at the site of a previous BCG vaccination.

11.5.3   Ophthalmic

Painless, nonexudative bilateral bulbar conjunctivitis may be associated with an iridocyclitis. It usually resolves rapidly and does not leave sequelae.

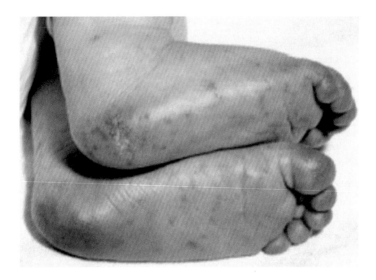

FIGURE 11.1 Desquamating rash in child with Kawasaki disease

11.5.4   Cardiovascular

Coronary aneurysms occur in up to 9 % of patients treated with IVIg in Japan. The coronary arteries are the most common site of aneurysm formation, but they can occur in any large artery (1 % of cases). Following treatment, the aneurysms may regress.

Valvular heart disease occurs in 1 % patients, with mitral regurgitation being the most common. The heart sounds may be faint, suggestive of pericardial effusion (Fig. 11.2). Pericarditis occurs in 13 % patients. A gallop rhythm is occasionally present.

11.6   Laboratory Features

There are no diagnostic tests for Kawasaki disease. The full blood count shows a neutrophilia and a thrombocytosis. The ESR and CRP are typically elevated. There can be a nonspecific transaminitis and urine analysis may show leucocytes and protein.

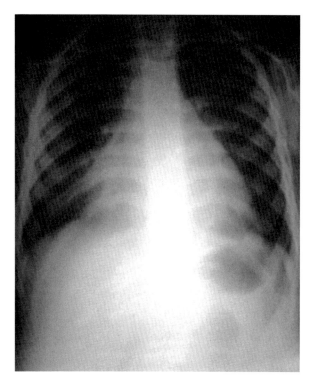

FIGURE 11.2 Chest X-ray showing enlarged in heart in child with Kawasaki disease

11.6.1   Radiology

A plain X-ray of the chest may demonstrate cardiomegaly (Fig. 11.2), but more importantly visible coronary artery calcification is a predictor of structural lesions [9].

11.6.2   Cardiac Investigations

Twelve-lead electrocardiography may show changes consistent with myocarditis or infarction (prolonged PR/QT intervals, abnormal Q waves, low voltage, ST-T changes), and dysrhythmias. 2D echocardiography is useful to show dilatation of coronary arteries, aneurysms, myocarditis, and pericardial effusions.

Coronary angiography enables accurate definition of coronary artery abnormalities and the severity of valvular lesions. Angiography should be performed in patients with cardiovascular involvement because there is a risk of progression to ischemic heart disease, especially in patients with giant aneurysms.

11.6.3   Immunology

Kawasaki disease is not associated with the presence of ANCA, RF, ANA, and anticardiolipin antibodies. Complement levels are normal.

11.6.4   Pathology

Coronary arteritis begins with oedema in the media with a lymphocytic and macrophage infiltration. This spreads to cause a panarteritis involving all layers of the vessel wall. Around the 12th day, the artery begins to dilate and abnormal blood flow leads to thrombus formation and vascular occlusion. Inflammatory cell infiltration continues for 3–4 weeks and then resolves, leaving scarring.

11.7   Diagnosis

There are no pathognomonic tests for the diagnosis of Kawasaki disease and pattern recognition is important. It is very important to recognize that there will be patients with incomplete Kawasaki disease in whom a diagnosis may have to be made without fulfilling all the criteria. Children with typical echocardiographic features can be labeled as having Kawasaki disease and should be treated as such in the absence of fulfilling other clinical criteria. Even for the purposes of classification, the criteria in Table 11.1 can be amended in the presence of coronary artery involvement (detected on echocardiography) and fever. In such a situation, the consensus view is that fewer than four of the remaining five criteria are sufficient, but the exact number of criteria required is yet to be determined.

The differential diagnosis includes erythema multiforme/ Stevens–Johnson syndrome, scarlet fever, toxic shock syndrome, systemic juvenile idiopathic arthritis, measles, and reactive arthritis.

11.8   Assessment of Disease Activity

Assessment of disease activity is clinical. Repeated echocardiography to note the progress or resolution of coronary arterial changes has been used in clinical trials. Coronary artery lumen corrected for the body surface area (Z score) has been used as an outcome measure in clinical trials. Resolution of clinical signs and acute phase reactions is expected with abatement of disease activity.

11.9   Treatment

A combination of aspirin and intravenous immunoglobulin is the mainstay of treatment of Kawasaki disease. Although there is a lack of clear trial evidence for the use of aspirin, it remains the standard of treatment in a dose of 100 mg/kg/day in four divided doses [10]. It is usual practice to reduce this dose to 3–5 mg/kg/day once the child is afebrile. Regular 2D echocardiograms may guide further use of aspirin. The aspirin can be stopped once the 2D echocardiogram normalizes. However, in children with persistent coronary arterial abnormalities, aspirin should be continued long-term. Intravenous immunoglobulin in a dose of 2 g/kg as a single infusion should be administered to all children, with a further dose of 2 g/kg in children who remain febrile 36 h after the first dose of immunoglobulin [7]. In children predicted to be refractory to intravenous immunoglobulin, the addition of prednisolone 2 mg/kg/day for 15 days after normalization of C-reactive protein reduces the risk of treatment failure and coronary artery lesions [11]. An alternative regimen of intravenous methylprednisolone 30 mg/kg/day for 1–3 days has also been used.

Other treatments used include pentoxifylline, plasmapheresis, cyclophosphomide and monoclonal antibodies like infliximab, abciximab, and etanercept.

11.10   Prognosis

Approximately 50 % of coronary arterial abnormalities regress within 5 years. However, giant aneurysms (more than 8 mm) are unlikely to resolve and may predispose to future risk of coronary thrombosis and myocardial infarction. The mortality is low (0.1–0.2 %) and is mainly due to myocardial infarction. In the past inflammatory response following Kawasaki disease was considered to be transient, but now it is recognized that markers of subclinical inflammation (serum amyloid A protein, high-sensitivity CRP) remain elevated years after clinical remission. These features may contribute directly to accelerated atherosclerosis. The 30 year survival rate for children suffering a myocardial infarction is 63 % [12]. The American Heart Association has recommended long-term treatment and further diagnostic testing according to risk stratification, dependent on the persistence and nature of coronary arterial involvement [13].

Key Points
- Kawasaki disease is an acute febrile illness involving the coronary circulation
- The diagnosis should be considered in any child with persisting fever, irrespective of the other clinical features
- Combination of intravenous immunoglobulin and aspirin is the mainstay of treatment
- Some children may go on to develop long-term coronary arterial problems which would need long-term care

References

1. Kato H, Koike S, Yamamoto M, Ito Y, Yano E. Coronary aneurysms in infants and young children with acute febrile mucocutaneous lymph node syndrome. J Pediatr. 1975;86(6):892–8.
2. Jennette JC, Falk RJ, Bacon PA, Basu N, Cid MC, Ferrario F, et al. 2012 revised International Chapel Hill Consensus Conference Nomenclature of Vasculitides. Arthritis Rheum. 2013;65(1):1–11.
3. Ozen S, Ruperto N, Dillon MJ, Bagga A, Barron K, Davin JC, et al. EULAR/PReS endorsed consensus criteria for the classification of childhood vasculitides. Ann Rheum Dis. 2006;65(7):936–41.
4. Nakamura Y, Yashiro M, Uehara R, Sadakane A, Tsuboi S, Aoyama Y, et al. Epidemiologic features of Kawasaki disease in Japan: results of the 2009–2010 nationwide survey. J Epidemiol. 2012;22(3):216–21.
5. Harnden A, Alves B, Sheikh A. Rising incidence of Kawasaki disease in England: analysis of hospital admission data. BMJ. 2002;324(7351):1424–5.
6. Lin YT, Manlhiot C, Ching JC, Han RK, Nield LE, Dillenburg R, et al. Repeated systematic surveillance of Kawasaki disease in Ontario from 1995 to 2006. Pediatr Int. 2010;52(5):699–706.
7. Singh S, Aulakh R. Kawasaki disease and Henoch Schonlein purpura: changing trends at a tertiary care hospital in north India (1993–2008). Rheumatol Int. 2010;30(6):771–4.
8. Burns JC, Herzog L, Fabri O, Tremoulet AH, Rodo X, Uehara R, et al. Seasonality of Kawasaki disease: a global perspective. PLoS One. 2013;8(9):e74529.
9. Lapierre C, Bitsch A, Guerin R, Garel L, Miro J, Dahdah N. Follow-up chest X-ray in patients with Kawasaki disease: the significance and clinical application of coronary artery macrocalcification. Pediatr Cardiol. 2010;31(1):56–61.
10. Baumer JH, Love SJ, Gupta A, Haines LC, Maconochie I, Dua JS. Salicylate for the treatment of Kawasaki disease in children. Cochrane Database Syst Rev. 2006;(4):CD004175.
11. Kobayashi T, Saji T, Otani T, Takeuchi K, Nakamura T, Arakawa H, et al. Efficacy of immunoglobulin plus prednisolone for prevention of coronary artery abnormalities in severe Kawasaki disease (RAISE study): a randomised, open-label, blinded-endpoints trial. Lancet. 2012;379(9826):1613–20.

12. Tsuda E, Hirata T, Matsuo O, Abe T, Sugiyama H, Yamada O. The 30-year outcome for patients after myocardial infarction due to coronary artery lesions caused by Kawasaki disease. Pediatr Cardiol. 2011;32(2):176–82.
13. Newburger JW, Takahashi M, Gerber MA, Gewitz MH, Tani LY, Burns JC, et al. Diagnosis, treatment, and long-term management of Kawasaki disease: a statement for health professionals from the Committee on Rheumatic Fever, Endocarditis, and Kawasaki Disease, Council on Cardiovascular Disease in the Young. American Heart Association. Pediatrics. 2004;114(6): 1708–33.

Chapter 12
IgA Vasculitis

12.1 Introduction

Schönlein and Henoch independently described a syndrome in children comprising joint pains, purpuric cutaneous lesions, abdominal colic, and malaena. Schönlein's description preceded the one by Henoch by about 40 years, and therefore, it is historically more accurate to term the syndrome Schönlein–Henoch purpura. William Heberden wrote about a child with arthralgia, edema, abdominal pain, vomiting, malaena, and purpura over the legs in 1801, 36 years prior to Schönlein. The eponym Henoch-Schönlein Purpura was abandoned in 2012, in favour of 'IgA vasculitis'.

12.2 Definition and Classification

The Chapel Hill Consensus Conference on the nomenclature of systemic vasculitis defined IgA vasculitis as "Vasculitis, with IgA1-dominant immune deposits, affecting small vessels (predominantly capillaries, venules, or arterioles). Often involves skin and gastrointestinal tract, and frequently causes arthritis. Glomerulonephritis indistinguishable from IgA nephropathy may occur" [1].

The ACR (1990) classification criteria (Table 12.1) have been widely used in clinical studies, but have relatively poor sensitivity (87.1 %) and specificity (87.7 %) [2]. These criteria

R.A. Watts et al., *Vasculitis in Clinical Practice*,
DOI 10.1007/978-3-319-14871-7_12,
© Springer International Publishing AG, Cham 2015

TABLE 12.1 ACR classification criteria for IgA vasculitis (Henoch–Schönlein purpura)

Palpable purpura

Slightly elevated purpuric rash over one or more areas of the skin not related to thrombocytopaenia

Bowel angina

Diffuse abdominal pain worse after meals, or bowel ischemia, usually bloody diarrhea

Age at onset <20 years

Development of first symptoms at age 20 years or less

Wall granulocytes on biopsy

Histological changes showing granulocytes in the walls of arteries or venules

From Mills et al. [2], with permission from John Wiley and Sons
Note that for purposes of classification, a patient shall be said to have IgA vasculitis if at least two of these four criteria are present

have recently been finalized for use in children by the European League Against Rheumatism, the Paediatric Rheumatology International Trials Organisation and the European Pediatric Rheumatology Society (Table 12.2) [3]. There are no validated diagnostic criteria.

12.3   Epidemiology

IgA vasculitis is a predominantly childhood vasculitic syndrome. It is the most common vasculitis in children and can occur from 6 months of age onward. Most of the children are less than 10 years of age. There is no obvious gender predisposition. The incidence of IgA vasculitis in adults is lower than in children, and in the UK, the incidence is 20.4/100,000 children [4], and 1.3/100,000 adults over the age of 16 years [5].

TABLE 12.2 EULAR/PRINTO/PReS classification criteria for childhood IgA vasculitis

Palpable purpura or petechiae (mandatory criterion) with lower limb predominance in the presence of at least one of the following four features:

Diffused abdominal pain

Any biopsy showing predominant IgA deposition

Arthritis[a] or arthralgia

Renal involvement (any hematuria and/or proteinuria)

From Ozen et al. [3], with permission from BMJ Publishing Group Ltd
[a]Acute, any joint

12.4   Etiology

The etiology of IgA vasculitis is unknown; however, there often appears to be a triggering upper respiratory infection especially in children. A number of drugs such as penicillin, erythromycin, and nonsteroidal anti-inflammatory drugs have been implicated as triggers.

12.5   Clinical Features

The classical features of IgA vasculitis are a triad of rash, gastrointestinal upset, and joint pain.

12.5.1   Cutaneous

The classical rash of IgA vasculitis is usually the first sign of the disease [6] (Figs. 12.1 and 12.2). It is an erythematous papular rash which develops into a palpable purpura. The usual distribution is on the dependent and pressure-bearing areas of the lower limbs and buttocks. The purpura may be preceded by an urticarial rash. The rash is usually symmetrical

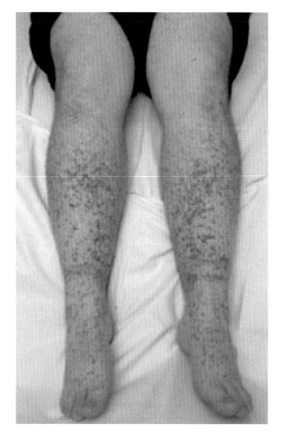

FIGURE 12.1 Purpuric lesions on the legs of a patient with Henoch–Schönlein purpura. Note the lesions along the pressure line caused by the patient's socks

and does not blanch with pressure. Skin necrosis may be seen in areas of severe cutaneous hemorrhage, and is more common in adults.

12.5.2   Gastrointestinal

The rash can be accompanied with gastrointestinal manifestations including abdominal pain, nausea, and vomiting. Abdominal pain is perhaps the second most frequent clinical

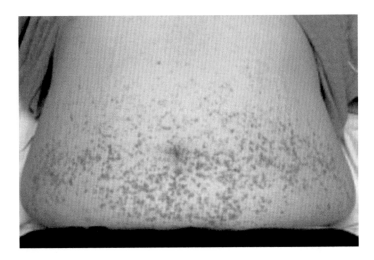

FIGURE 12.2 Purpuric lesions on the abdomen in a patient with Henoch–Schönlein purpura

manifestation after the skin rash. It is frequently colicky, and the severity may wax and wane in relation with new crops of skin lesions. The pain is thought to be due to submucosal hemorrhages. These can produce GI bleeds which can manifest as hematemesis or malaena. Infrequently acute intussusception has been observed in children.

12.5.3   Musculoskeletal

Arthralgia is a common manifestation and can precede the development of palpable purpura by several days. Joint pains with or without obvious synovitis usually involves the lower limbs. Arthralgia is usually transient and does not leave any long-term sequelae.

12.5.4   Renal

Renal involvement includes a spectrum of severity extending from asymptomatic hematuria and mild proteinuria to glomerulonephritis accompanied by hypertension and

elevated serum creatinine. The most severe clinical manifestation is probably the mixed nephritic/nephrotic picture
with hematuria, hypertension, elevated serum creatinine,
severe proteinuria, and hypoalbuminemia. The renal
involvement of Henoch–Schönlein purpura is perhaps the
most common manifestation responsible for the chronicity
of the disease. The frequency of renal involvement is pro-
portionally much higher in adults (80 %) than in children
(33 %).

Neurological

Central and peripheral nervous system is uncommon but well
documented [7]. Altered consciousness, convulsions, focal
neurological deficits, visual abnormalities and verbal disability may be seen from central nervous lesions due to intrace-
rebral haemorrhage, posterior subcortical oedema, sagittal
sinus thrombosis or diffuse cerebral oedema. Facial palsy,
acute demyelinating polyneuropathy, brachial plexopathy,
ulnar neuropathy, femoral neuropathy, posterior tibial neuropathy or peroneal neuropathy may be manifestations of
peripheral nervous involvement.

12.6   Laboratory Features

The inflammatory markers are almost always elevated. The
full blood count shows leucocytosis and thrombocytosis in
the acute phase of the disease. A low hemoglobin may be a
sign of a gastrointestinal bleed.

12.6.1   Renal Function

Urine may be positive for RBCs, leucocytes, and protein.
Microscopy may reveal red cell casts in the presence of glo-
merulonephritis. Renal function should be quantified with
GFR, together with an estimation of urine protein leak.

12.6.2   Immunology

The serum IgA levels may be increased. Serological tests such as ANA, ANCA, RF, and anticardiolipin antibodies should all be negative. A positive ANA or ANCA should prompt an assessment for systemic vasculitis or SLE.

12.6.3   Pathology

The cutaneous lesions of IgA vasculitis show a small vessel vasculitis with the involvement of the capillaries, post capillary venules, and nonmuscular arteries. Often there is leucocytoclasis (Fig. 12.3). The appearances are difficult to distinguish from leucocytoclastic (hypersensitivity) vasculitis or other small vessel vasculitis. IgA deposits are present in the skin lesions of IgA vasculitis and may be a distinguishing feature.

A renal biopsy should be considered in both children and adults, if there is significant proteinuria or hematuria which

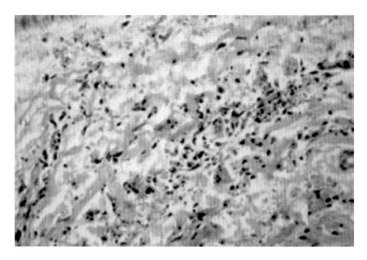

FIGURE 12.3 Skin biopsy showing leucocytoclasis in a patient with IgA vasculitis

persists. In the kidney, the earliest lesion is a focal or diffuse proliferative glomerulonephritis. The appearances may be indistinguishable from IgA nephropathy. Immunofluorescence reveals diffuse mesangial IgA deposition.

12.7   Diagnosis

The diagnosis of IgA vasculitis should be suspected in children and adults who have purpuric lesions involving the lower limbs, with or without arthralgia, abdominal pain, or renal involvement. The diagnosis is confirmed with the classical histopathological picture. There is no absolute diagnostic test, and the criteria in Tables 12.1 and 12.2 are classification criteria used for academic purposes. Other conditions, which can mimic IgA vasculitis, are drug-induced vasculitis, and infections (especially *Neiserria meningitides*) and idiopathic thrombocytopenic purpura.

12.8   Assessment of Disease Activity

The Birmingham Vasculitis Activity Score v3 and the Disease Extent Index have both been validated for assessing disease severity in IgA vasculitis [8]. The inflammatory markers in acute phase reactions usually follow the waxing and waning of the rash. Children with renal involvement can continue to have microscopic hematuria and mild proteinuria long after the acute phase of the disease. This does not necessarily need escalation of treatment.

12.9   Treatment

Most children and adults with IgA vasculitis do not need any specific treatment. Treatment with nonsteroidal anti-inflammatory agents is usually sufficient for the arthralgia.

This should be avoided in patients with a gastrointestinal bleed. There is no evidence for the use of glucocorticoid therapy, but anecdotally adult patients more often require glucocorticoids. In children, several RCTs have shown that the routine use of glucocorticoids does not alter the progression to severe nephritis or GI involvement [9, 10]. The acute hypertension may need treatment with an antihypertensive. Patients with acute renal failure will need renal supportive treatment. There are no large RCTs to guide therapy in patients with rapidly progressive or established glomerulonephritis; such patients should be treated with glucocorticoids and immunosuppressants. There is limited evidence for the role of cyclosporine A in childhood renal involvement [11], and leflunomide in adult renal involvement [12].

Glucocorticoids are effective in reducing the severity of abdominal pain and arthralgias. Intussusception should be excluded first.

12.10 Prognosis

Most children and adults with IgA vasculitis have a self-limiting disease within 2–3 weeks. However, the disease has been known to relapse in about 50 % of children and a small proportion of these patients go on to develop chronic vasculitic syndrome. The long-term morbidity and mortality of HSP patients are predominantly related to the level of renal involvement. Children presenting with acute nephritic syndrome have a less favorable outcome with a long-term risk of chronic renal failure, but those with a mixed nephritic/nephrotic presentation have the worst long-term outcome with up to a third developing chronic renal failure. Overall, <5 % of children develop chronic renal failure. Renal failure is more common in adults. In transplanted patients, renal graft survival is 80 % at 5 years and just under 60 % at 10 years [13]. Recurrent disease causing graft failure occurs in about 14 % of patients.

Key Points
- Henoch–Schönlein purpura is mainly a vasculitic syndrome of childhood.
- It is usually self-limiting, but in a small proportion of patients, especially those with renal involvement and a mixed nephritic/nephrotic picture, develop chronic renal failure and long-term sequelae.
- There is no specific treatment for Henoch–Schönlein purpura and most cases need only supportive treatment and nonsteroidal anti-inflammatory drugs.

References

1. Jennette JC, Falk RJ, Bacon PA, Basu N, Cid MC, Ferrario F, et al. 2012 revised International Chapel Hill Consensus Conference Nomenclature of Vasculitides. Arthritis Rheum. 2013;65(1):1–11.
2. Mills JA, Michel BA, Bloch DA, Calabrese LH, Hunder GG, Arend WP, et al. The American College of Rheumatology 1990 criteria for the classification of Henoch-Schonlein purpura. Arthritis Rheum. 1990;33(8):1114–21.
3. Ozen S, Pistorio A, Iusan SM, Bakkaloglu A, Herlin T, Brik R, et al. EULAR/PRINTO/PRES criteria for Henoch-Schonlein purpura, childhood polyarteritis nodosa, childhood Wegener granulomatosis and childhood Takayasu arteritis: Ankara 2008. Part II: Final classification criteria. Ann Rheum Dis. 2010; 69(5):798–806.
4. Gardner-Medwin JM, Dolezalova P, Cummins C, Southwood TR. Incidence of Henoch-Schonlein purpura, Kawasaki disease, and rare vasculitides in children of different ethnic origins. Lancet. 2002;360(9341):1197–202.
5. Watts RA, Jolliffe VA, Grattan CE, Elliott J, Lockwood M, Scott DG. Cutaneous vasculitis in a defined population–clinical and epidemiological associations. J Rheumatol. 1998;25(5):920–4.
6. Saulsbury FT. Henoch-Schonlein purpura in children. Report of 100 patients and review of the literature. Medicine (Baltimore). 1999;78(6):395–409.

7. Garzoni L, Vanoni F, Rizzi M, Simonetti GD, Goeggel Simonetti B, Ramelli GP, et al. Nervous system dysfunction in Henoch-Schonlein syndrome: systematic review of the literature. Rheumatology (Oxford). 2009;48(12):1524–9.

8. Demirkaya E, Ozen S, Pistorio A, Galasso R, Ravelli A, Hasija R, et al. Performance of Birmingham Vasculitis Activity Score and disease extent index in childhood vasculitides. Clin Exp Rheumatol. 2012;30(1 Suppl 70):S162–8.

9. Ronkainen J, Koskimies O, Ala-Houhala M, Antikainen M, Merenmies J, Rajantie J, et al. Early prednisone therapy in Henoch-Schonlein purpura: a randomized, double-blind, placebo-controlled trial. J Pediatr. 2006;149(2):241–7.

10. Huber AM, King J, McLaine P, Klassen T, Pothos M. A randomized, placebo-controlled trial of prednisone in early Henoch Schonlein Purpura [ISRCTN85109383]. BMC Med. 2004;2:7.

11. Jauhola O, Ronkainen J, Autio-Harmainen H, Koskimies O, Ala-Houhala M, Arikoski P, et al. Cyclosporine A vs. methylprednisolone for Henoch-Schonlein nephritis: a randomized trial. Pediatr Nephrol. 2011;26(12):2159–66.

12. Zhang Y, Gao Y, Zhang Z, Liu G, He H, Liu L. Leflunomide in addition to steroids improves proteinuria and renal function in adult Henoch-Schoenlein nephritis with nephrotic proteinuria. Nephrology (Carlton). 2014;19(2):94–100.

13. Samuel JP, Bell CS, Molony DA, Braun MC. Long-term outcome of renal transplantation patients with Henoch-Schonlein purpura. Clin J Am Soc Nephrol. 2011;6(8):2034–40.

Chapter 13
Behçet's Disease

13.1 Introduction

Hulusi Behçet, a dermato-venerologist in Istanbul, described three patients with oral aphthous and genital ulceration along with hypopyon uveitis in 1937. Although he is honored with the eponymous syndrome, it may have been first described in Hippocrates' third book of endemic diseases in fifth century BC. Benedictos Adamantiades, a Greek ophthalmologist, independently described the syndrome in 1930, and the disease is known as Adamantiades–Behçet's syndrome in some parts of the world.

13.2 Definition and Classification

There is no recognized definition of this condition. It is generally recognized to be a triad of anterior uveitis usually resulting in a hypopyon, oral aphthous ulceration, and genital ulceration. The International Study Group (ISG) diagnostic criteria are widely used, but have not been formally validated (Table 13.1) [1]. The International Criteria for Behcet's disease (ICBD) have recently proposed and validated an alternative criteria which are more sensitive but less specific to the ISG criteria (Table 13.2) [2].

R.A. Watts et al., *Vasculitis in Clinical Practice*,
DOI 10.1007/978-3-319-14871-7_13,
© Springer International Publishing AG, Cham 2015

TABLE 13.1 International Study Group diagnostic (classification) criteria for Behçet's syndrome (1990)

Criteria	Definition
Recurrent oral ulceration	Minor aphthous, major aphthous, or herpetiform ulceration observed by physician or patient recurring at least three times in one 12-month period
Plus two of	
Recurrent genital ulceration	Aphthous ulceration or scarring, observed by physician or patient
Eye lesions	Anterior uveitis, posterior uveitis, cells in the vitreous on slit-lamp examination, or retinal vasculitis observed by ophthalmologist
Skin lesions	Erythema nodosum observed by physician or patient, pseudofolliculitis, papulopustular lesions, or acneiform nodules observed by physician in postadolescent patients not on corticosteroids treatment
Pathergy	Read by physician at 24–48 h

Adapted from [1]

TABLE 13.2 International criteria for Behcet's disease (2014)

Criteria	Points
Eye lesions	2 points
Oral aphthosis	2 points
Genital aphthosis	2 points
Skin lesions	1 point
CNS involvement	1 point
Pathergy	1 point

A score of ≥4 points is 95 % sensitive and 90 % specific for classification of Behcet's disease [2]

13.3 Epidemiology

Behçet's disease is also known as the 'silk route disease' due to its geographical distribution along the overland trading routes from the Far East to Europe by way of the Middle East and the Mediterranean. The prevalence of Behçet's disease in Turkey is thought to be between 80 and 420 per 100,000 [3]. Behçet's disease is uncommon in the UK and Northern Europe. The prevalence in Sweden is 4.9 per 100,000 [4]. The usual onset is in the third decade, and although childhood Behçet's disease has been described, it is rare even in the Mediterranean. There is preponderance of the disease in males. No environmental factors have been associated with Behçet's disease.

13.4 Etiology

The etiology of Behçet's disease is unknown, but it is not felt to have an autoimmune pathogenesis. Autoantibodies are not generally found in Behçet's disease. There is strong association with HLA-B51.

13.5 Clinical Features

The initial symptoms can be nonspecific. BD is a multisystem disease and not all features are apparent at presentation, and therefore, a detailed history with special regard to orogenital ulceration is needed.

13.5.1 Orogenital

Recurrent oral ulceration is usually the first symptom and most patients will have ulceration at some stage of their

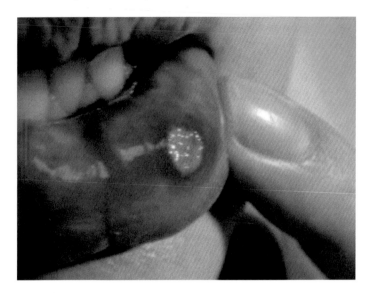

FIGURE 13.1 Oral ulceration in Behçet's disease

disease. The ulcers are usually <10 mm in diameter, although the ulcers can be much bigger and herpetiform (Fig. 13.1). They start as erythematous raised circular areas, which develop into circular areas of ulceration. The ulcers have a gray pseudomembrane and surrounding erythema. They are usually localized over the mucosal surfaces, but infrequently can affect the hard palate, tonsils, and pharynx. Major aphthae can heal with scarring, but this rarely causes significant compromise of deglutition.

Genital ulceration in males is usually scrotal, and infrequently, on the shaft or on the glans penis. In females, the labia majora and minora can be ulcerated. The ulcers usually commence as papules or pustules, which rapidly ulcerate. The ulcers have a punched-out appearance. They can be larger, more painful, and deeper than the oral ulcers. Genital ulcers are resistant to treatment, more likely to get infected, and usually heal with scarring.

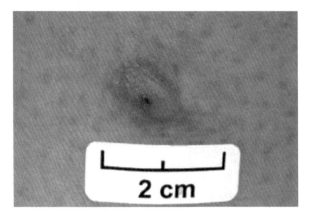

FIGURE 13.2 Pathergy test in Behçet's disease – pustule induced by a dermal puncture with a 20G needle

13.5.2   Cutaneous

Other skin lesions seen in Behçet's disease include erythema nodosum, superficial thrombophlebitis, and pyoderma gangrenosum. Acne-like papulopustular lesions are commonly present at the usual areas of acne such as the face, upper chest, and back, but they are only of cosmetic concern. A papulopustular reaction within 48 h of a needle prick is seen in some patients and is termed "pathergy." This is characteristic of Behçet's disease and a papulopustular reaction to dermal puncture with a 20G needle has been used for diagnostic purposes (Fig. 13.2). Neutrophilic dermatosis (Sweet's syndrome) has been reported in Behçet's disease.

13.5.3   Ophthalmic

The involvement is in the form of panuveitis and retinal vasculitis. The presence of a layer of pus in the anterior chamber (hypopyon) suggests intense inflammation and is associated with an adverse prognosis (Fig. 13.3). Eye involve-

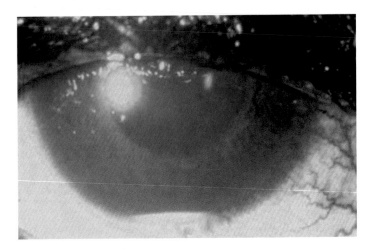

FIGURE 13.3 Hypopyon in Behçet's disease

ment is frequently bilateral and appears early within the first few years of the disease. It is rare for individuals to develop *de novo* eye involvement after the first 5 years [5]. Visual acuity at presentation is worse than 20/40 in 50 %, and 20/200 or worse in 21 % of affected eyes [6]. Recurrent disease flares in the eye result in secondary changes such as cataracts and glaucoma due to the formation of synechiae. Ocular inflammation can continue even after global eye atrophy. Enucleation of the affected eye may be the only way of controlling disease activity in those patients. The common symptoms of eye disease are blurred vision, periorbital pain, photophobia, scleral injection, and excessive lacrimation.

13.5.4 *Neurological*

Neurological involvement is reported between 5 and 50 %, but when it occurs, is usually the most serious aspect of the disease. There are two main causes for neurological manifestations in Behçet's disease – parenchymal involvement and venous sinus thrombosis. Demyelination is the usual cause of the neurological manifestations, but encephalomalacia and cerebral atrophy are also seen. Anatomically, the most common site of involvement is the brain stem, followed by the spinal cord, cerebrum, and cerebellum. Neurological involvement is a late feature occurring 1–8 years after disease onset. Individuals present with evidence of pyramidal tract involvement, headache, ataxia, or sensory involvement. Less commonly, they may present with features of dementia, aseptic meningitis, or involuntary movements.

13.5.5   Vascular

Behçet's disease can involve any part of the vascular tree – aortitis, pulmonary arterial involvement, medium-sized vessel involvement, leukocytoclastic vasculitis, portal vein thrombosis, deep venous thrombosis, dural sinus thrombosis are all a feature of Behçet's disease. Clinical manifestations will vary depending on the site of the lesions. Large vessel disease is commoner in males. Behçet's disease is one of the few differentials for pulmonary arterial aneurysms. Pulmonary vasculature involvement is rare affecting 1.5–7.5 %, but can be fatal. Patients with pulmonary arterial aneurysms can present with pulmonary hemorrhage. Occlusive disease of the major arteries of the lower limbs, renal involvement, cerebral vessel involvement, and myocardial involvement has all been documented. Major vascular involvement is associated with constitutional symptoms such as fever and weight loss.

13.5.6   Musculoskeletal

A nonerosive, asymmetric, large joint oligoarthropathy usually involving joints of the lower limbs may occur. Avascular necrosis unrelated to the use of glucocorticoid therapy can develop.

13.5.7   Gastrointestinal

Mucosal ulceration may involve any part of the intestinal tract, colitis, esophageal ulceration, and portal vein thrombosis. The lesion may be indistinguishable from those occurring in inflammatory bowel disease.

13.5.8   Renal

A nephritic syndrome may occur due to the disease. In long standing cases, a nephrotic syndrome due to amyloidosis has been observed.

13.6   Laboratory Features

The CRP and ESR may be elevated during an acute attack. There may be an anemia of chronic disease, neutrophilia; thrombocytosis may be present in active disease. The alkaline phosphatase may be elevated in some patients.

13.6.1   Immunology

Immunology tests such as ANCA, ANA RF, and anticardiolipin antibodies are usually negative. IgA levels may be elevated.

13.6.2   Genetic

HLA B51 has been associated with Behçet's disease, but its absence does not rule out the diagnosis.

13.6.3   Synovial Fluid Examination

Synovial fluid analysis reveals the presence of leucocytes, without crystals or microorganisms.

13.6.4   Cerebrospinal Fluid

The CSF shows pleocytosis, elevated protein levels, low normal glucose levels.

13.6.5   Imaging

Imaging of the head is useful in diagnosis and follow-up of patients with neurological involvement. Dural sinus thrombosis, meningeal involvement, cerebral atrophy, demyelination, and small vessel ischemic changes can all be demonstrated on computed tomography or magnetic resonance imaging of the head. Digital subtraction angiography or other forms of angiography can be used to demonstrate large vessel stenosis or aneurysms.

13.6.6   Pathology

Biopsy of the oral and genital ulcers shows lymphocytic and monocytic inflammatory infiltrate in the basal layer and dermis with erosion of the epidermis. Leukocytoclastic vasculitis may be observed. None of these laboratory features are specific for the diagnosis of Behçet's disease.

13.7   Diagnosis

There are no diagnostic criteria for the Behçet's disease. Diagnosis is mainly on clinical grounds. Diagnosis may be delayed in patients who have recurrent oral ulceration without development of other features for years. The differential diagnosis is from other types of vasculitis. The key feature is the presence of orogenital ulcers as there are few other conditions in which this is a predominant feature. Oral ulcers need to be differentiated from other types of ulcers such as benign aphthous ulcers, viral infection, and inflammatory bowel disease. The oral ulcers of BD tend to be more frequent and multiple. The genital ulcers need to be differentiated from herpetic ulcers and other viral ulcers or inflammatory bowel disease. The MAGIC syndrome is an overlap between relapsing polychondritis and BD. Mouth and genital ulcers with inflamed cartilage (MAGIC).

13.8   Assessment of Disease Activity

There are no valid biomarkers for the assessment of disease activity in Behçet's disease. Aphthous ulcer count, time to healing, MR imaging of the brain, visual acuity, and visual analog scales for pain, have all been used as outcome measures in clinical trials. A patient reported outcome measure – Behcet's Syndrome Activity Score (BSAS) has been validated in Turkish patients as a measure of disease activity [7]. Practically, the progress is largely based on clinical examination and symptomatology assisted by change in the acute phase reactants (if they were abnormal to begin with).

13.9   Treatment

Management depends on the nature of the manifestations. Treatment is dictated by the clinically dominant lesion [8].

13.9.1   Mucocutaneous

In isolated oral or genital ulcers, the first-line of treatment should be topical treatments (anesthetic gels, glucocorticoids, sucralfate). Colchicine is useful in patients with erythema nodosum. Patients with resistant mucosal ulceration may be treated with azathioprine or colchicine. Thalidomide has been recommended in refractory cases, but it has to be used with care in women in the child bearing age group. Interferon alpha and tumor necrosis factor alpha have been recommended in the most extreme cases. Acneiform lesions need symptomatic treatment only.

13.9.2   Ocular

Posterior uveitis must be treated with a combination of azathioprine 2.5 mg/kg/day and topical or systemic glucocorticoid therapy. Azathioprine prevents relapses and is advocated long-term in this group of patients. Patients with retinal disease and severe eye disease (>2 lines drop in visual acuity on a 10/10 scale) should have ciclosporine A 2–5 mg/kg/day or infliximab in combination with azathioprine and glucocorticoid. For patients who cannot tolerate this combination, interferon alpha ± glucocorticoid can be used as second-line. Adalimumab has been used with success in patients refractory to infliximab [9].

13.9.3   Vasculopathy

Patients with large vessel vasculopathy should be treated with a combination of cyclophosphamide and glucocorticoid therapy. Patients with deep venous thrombosis should receive azathioprine or cyclophosphamide or ciclosporine A or glucocorticoids, instead of anticoagulation. Deep vein thrombi in Behçet's disease are adherent to the vessel wall and do not embolize. There is no advantage in offering routing anticoagulation to these patients, but immunosuppression is associated with a lower risk of relapse of venous thrombosis [10]. Immunosuppression should also be offered or continued in patients undergoing vascular surgery [11].

13.9.4   Gastrointestinal

There is no evidence base for the management of gastrointestinal involvement. However, azathioprine may be tried with glucocorticoid therapy.

13.9.5 Musculoskeletal

Arthritis of Behçet's disease is nonerosive and generally wellcontrolled with colchicine 1–2 mg/day. Intramuscular depot methylprednisolone is not effective. Resistant cases may be treated with interferon alpha, azathioprine, or tumor necrosis factor alpha blockade.

13.9.6 Neurological

Neurological involvement must be treated with pulsed intravenous methylprednisolone 1 g/day for 3–7 days followed by the maintenance of oral prednisolone tapered over 2–3 months. Interferon alpha and tumor necrosis factor alpha blockade have been used with some benefit in resistant cases. Patients with dural venous thrombosis should be treated with a brief course of glucocorticoid therapy. Ciclosporine A is neurotoxic and should be avoided in patients with neurological involvement, unless the dominant manifestation is ocular and they cannot tolerate infliximab.

13.10   Prognosis

Young males with Behçet's disease have a poor prognosis. In a 20-year survey, males between 14 and 24 years of age had a standardized mortality ratio of 13.36 (95 % confidence interval 4.90, 29.08) [5]. Patients with eye disease, vascular disease, and neurological involvement are statistically more likely to have an adverse prognosis [5]. The presence of HLA-B51 adversely affects functional outcomes and survival [12]. With increasing age, Behçet's seems to become quiescent, with the exception of neurological involvement and large vessel disease, which present later in the disease. About a fifth of patients with Behçet's disease suffer significant impairment of vision. This has improved in recent times, perhaps due to early recognition and earlier use of immunosuppressive therapy. The arthritis is usually self-limiting, nonerosive, and responsive to short courses of glucocorticoid therapy or colchicine.

Key Points

- Behçet's disease is a multisystem disease with vasculitis, which can affect any part of the vasculature.
- Most of the patients will have a history of recurrent oral ulceration or genital ulceration.
- There are no diagnostic criteria, validated biomarkers, or laboratory tests to assist diagnosis or monitoring, which is purely on clinical grounds.
- Neurological involvement and large vessel vasculitis are uncommon features, but account for most of the mortality due to Behçet's disease.
- Treatment of Behçet's disease is dependent on the manifestation. It has a poor evidence base due to the rarity of the condition.

References

1. Criteria for diagnosis of Behcet's disease. International Study Group for Behcet's Disease. Lancet. 1990;335(8697):1078–80.
2. International Team for the Revision of the International Criteria for Behçet's Disease (ITR-ICBD). The International Criteria for Behçet's Disease (ICBD): a collaborative study of 27 countries on the sensitivity and specificity of the new criteria. J Eur Acad Dermatol Venereol. 2014;28(3):338–47.
3. Yurdakul S, Yazici H. Behcet's syndrome. Best Pract Res Clin Rheumatol. 2008;22(5):793–809.
4. Mohammad A, Mandl T, Sturfelt G, Segelmark M. Incidence, prevalence and clinical characteristics of Behçet's disease in southern Sweden. Rheumatology (Oxford). 2013;52(2):304–10.
5. Kural-Seyahi E, Fresko I, Seyahi N, Ozyazgan Y, Mat C, Hamuryudan V, et al. The long-term mortality and morbidity of Behcet syndrome: a 2-decade outcome survey of 387 patients

followed at a dedicated center. Medicine (Baltimore). 2003;82(1):60–76.

6. Taylor SR, Singh J, Menezo V, Wakefield D, McCluskey P, Lightman S. Behcet disease: visual prognosis and factors influencing the development of visual loss. Am J Ophthalmol. 2011;152(6):1059–66.

7. Yilmaz S, Simsek I, Cinar M, Erdem H, Kose O, Yazici Y, et al. Patient-driven assessment of disease activity in Behcet's syndrome: cross-cultural adaptation, reliability and validity of the Turkish version of the Behcet's Syndrome Activity Score. Clin Exp Rheumatol. 2013;31(3 Suppl 77):77–83.

8. Hatemi G, Silman A, Bang D, Bodaghi B, Chamberlain AM, Gul A, et al. EULAR recommendations for the management of Behcet disease. Ann Rheum Dis. 2008;67(12):1656–62.

9. Perra D, Alba MA, Callejas JL, Mesquida M, Rios-Fernandez R, Adan A, et al. Adalimumab for the treatment of Behcet's disease: experience in 19 patients. Rheumatology (Oxford). 2012;51(10):1825–31.

10. Desbois AC, Wechsler B, Resche-Rigon M, Piette JC, Huong Dle T, Amoura Z, et al. Immunosuppressants reduce venous thrombosis relapse in Behcet's disease. Arthritis Rheum. 2012;64(8):2753–60.

11. Ha YJ, Jung SY, Lee KH, Jung SJ, Lee SW, Park MC, et al. Long-term clinical outcomes and risk factors for the occurrence of post-operative complications after cardiovascular surgery in patients with Behcet's disease. Clin Exp Rheumatol. 2012;30(3 Suppl 72):S18–26.

12. Noel N, Bernard R, Wechsler B, Resche-Rigon M, Depaz R, Le Thi Huong Boutin D, et al. Long-term outcome of neuro-Behcet's disease. Arthritis Rheumatol. 2014;66(5):1306–14.

Chapter 14
Cryoglobulinemic Vasculitis

14.1 Introduction

Cryoglobulinemic vasculitis is a rare medium/small vessel vasculitis that is often associated with Hepatitis C virus (HCV) infection.

14.2 Definition

The Chapel Hill Consensus Conference defined cryoglobulinemic vasculitis as vasculitis, with cryoglobulin immune deposits, affecting small vessels (predominately capillaries, venules, or arterioles), and associated with cryoglobulins in serum. Skin and glomeruli are often involved [1].

14.3 Epidemiology

The epidemiology of cryoglobulinemic vasculitis has not been well described. It appears to be more common in areas with high rates of HCV infection especially Southern Europe compared with Northern Europe or the USA. The condition is more common in women than in men (3:1).

R.A. Watts et al., *Vasculitis in Clinical Practice*,
DOI 10.1007/978-3-319-14871-7_14,
© Springer International Publishing AG, Cham 2015

14.4   Etiology

HCV was first identified in 1989. There is a strong association between HCV infection and essential mixed cryoglobuline-mia, with 80–90 % of such patients being positive for anti-HCV antibodies. Circulating HCV-RNA has been identified in the peripheral blood of patients with cryoglobulinemia. HCV has been identified within cutaneous vasculitic lesions and has been selectively concentrated together with specific antibody in cryoprecipitates.

14.5   Clinical Features

In the early stages, the symptoms can be nonspecific and a high index of suspicion is required to achieve an early diag-nosis. Meltzer's triad (purpura, arthralgia, weakness) occurs in <40 % of patients [2].

14.5.1   Systemic

A constitutional illness with fever, weight loss, myalgia, arthralgia commonly occurs.

14.5.2   Cutaneous

The most typical feature is a purpuric rash. Less common features include urticaria, livedo, exanthem, acral necrosis, and leg ulcers. Raynaud's phenomenon occurs in 20 %.

14.5.3   Neurological

Polyneuropathy is present in 40–70 % (distal, symmetrical or asymmetrical, motor and/or sensory polyneuropathy, acute mononeuritis multiplex). Mononeuritis multiple is typically of acute onset. Peripheral neuropathy is typically of subacute gradual onset.

14.5.4   Renal

Renal involvement (nephrotic syndrome or nephritic urinary sediment due to mesangial proliferative glomerulonephritis occurs in <40 %.

14.5.5   Musculoskeletal

Arthralgias or arthritis occur in 10 % and is not erosive.

14.6   Laboratory Features

Cryoglobulins are cold insoluble immune complexes containing rheumatoid factor, polyclonal IgG, and HCV RNA that precipitate and deposit on vascular endothelium (Fig. 14.1). They arise from the development of clonal expansion of rheumatoid factor-expressing B cells in liver, lymph nodes and peripheral blood. Cryoglobulins may be detected in peripheral blood or in tissue biopsies especially renal biopsy specimens. Peripheral blood samples for cryoglobulin detection must be kept warm during transport to the laboratory.

14.6.1   Viral Serology

HCV is present in >90 % of cases of cryoglobulinemic vasculitis. Serology for other potential viral causes of vasculitis (e.g., HBV, HIV and CMV) should be performed.

14.6.2   Immunology

Rheumatoid factor in high titres are present in 70 %, however ANCA, ANA, anticardiolipin antibodies are typically negative. Hypocomplementemia is present in 90 % of cases.

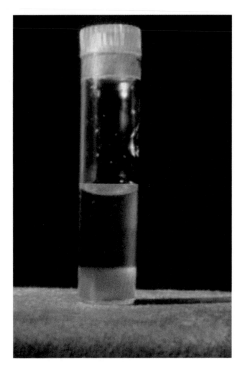

FIGURE 14.1 Cryoprecipitate from a patient with cryoglobulinemia

14.6.3   Pathology

The characteristic lesion on renal biopsy is a membranopro-
liferative glomerulonephritis with intracapillary thrombi,
which contain cryoglobulin precipitates. This distinguishes it
from ANCA-associated vasculitis in which a focal segmental
necrotizing glomerulonephritis is the typical lesion.

14.7   Diagnosis

The differential diagnosis is from other types of systemic vasculitis. The diagnosis is usually made with viral serology
together with appropriate tissue biopsy. Hypocomplementemia

is a useful distinguishing feature from most other types of vasculitis, especially ANCA-associated vasculitis in which complement levels are normal.

14.8   Assessment of Disease Activity

Individual organ involvement should be assessed. In patients suspected of a systemic vasculitis urinalysis (looking for proteinuria, hematuria, red cell casts) should be performed urgently. Renal function should be assessed by creatinine clearance, quantification of protein leak if present using either 24 h protein excretion or urine protein/creatinine ratio.

14.9   Treatment

Treatment may target either the viral trigger (HCV) or the subsequent B cell mediated autoimmunity.

The use of anti-viral therapy in the treatment of cryoglobulinemic vasculitis was recommended in the EULAR guidelines for the management of medium/small vessel vasculitis [3].

Antiviral therapy is with pegylated-IFN alpha plus ribavirin. Ribavirin alone is ineffective and should not be used. Two recent prospective randomized controlled trials investigated the role of rituximab in patients in whom anti-viral therapy had failed to induce remission. The studies demonstrated that rituximab monotherapy was superior to conventional immunosuppression using corticlsteroids, azathioprine, cyclophosphamide, methotrexate or plasmapheresis [4, 5].

14.10   Prognosis

The prognosis is determined by age, severity of renal involvement and extent of vasculitis.

Key Points
- Cryoglobulinemic vasculitis is usually associated with HCV infection.
- Meltzer's triad (purpura, arthralgia, weakness) occurs in <40 % of patients.
- Treatment for most patients is with pegylated IFN-alpha, and ribavirin.

References

1. Jennette JC, Falk RJ, Bacon PA, et al. 2012 revised International Chapel Hill Consensus Conference nomenclature of vasculitides. Arthritis Rheum. 2013;65:1–11.
2. Ramos-Casals M, Stone JH, Cid MC, Bosch X. The cryoglobu-linaemias. Lancet. 2012;379:348–60.
3. Mukhtyar C, Guillevin L, Cid M, et al. EULAR recommendations for the management of primary small and medium vasculitis. Ann Rheum Dis. 2009;68:310–7.
4. De Vita S, Quartuccio L, Isola M, et al. A randomized controlled trial of rituximab for the treatment of severe cryoglobulinaemic vasculitis. Arthritis Rheum. 2012;64:843–53.
5. Sneller MC, Hu Z, Langford CA. A randomized controlled trial of rituximab following failure of antiviral therapy for hepatitis C virus associated cryoglobulinaemic vasculitis. Arthritis Rheum. 2012;64:835–42.

Chapter 15
Vasculitis Mimics

15.1 Introduction

The presenting features of the systemic vasculitides are protean and diagnosis is based on a combination of clinical, laboratory and histopathological features. Clinical features alone are not always diagnostic as a variety of other diseases can mimic systemic vasculitis (Table 15.1). These mimics usually present with multiorgan illness or evidence of vascular damage, or a combination of both. Biopsy of involved organs is, therefore, important to identify noninflammatory vascular changes such as embolism or thrombosis. For example, angiographic features including aneurysms, though typical of PAN, can occur in other conditions such as myxoma and bacterial endocarditis.

15.2 Cholesterol Crystal Embolism

Cholesterol crystal embolism has been recognized for more than a century; however, it remains under diagnosed and is sometimes called "trash foot." Risk factors for cholesterol embolism are male gender, age >60 years, Caucasian ethnicity, hypertension, tobacco use, and diabetes mellitus [1]. Cholesterol embolism may occur spontaneously or after trauma to the aortic wall during vascular surgery including

R.A. Watts et al., *Vasculitis in Clinical Practice*,
DOI 10.1007/978-3-319-14871-7_15,
© Springer International Publishing AG, Cham 2015

TABLE 15.1 Vasculitis mimics

Systemic multisystem disease	
Infection	Subacute bacterial endocarditis
	Neisseria
	Rickettsiae
Malignancy	Metastatic carcinoma
Paraneoplastic	
Other	Sweet syndrome
	Scurvy
	Cocaine abuse
Occlusive vasculopathy	
Embolic	Cholesterol crystals
	Atrial myxoma
	Infection
Thrombotic	Antiphospholipid syndrome
	Procoagulant states
	Calciphylaxis
Others	Ergot
	Radiation
	Köhlmeier–Degos
	Severe Raynaud's
	Acute digital loss
Angiographic	
Aneurysmal	Fibromuscular dysplasia
	Neurofibromatosis
Occlusion	Coarctation

endovascular or angiographic procedures. Other etiological factors include anticoagulation therapy with either heparin or warfarin and thrombolysis [2]. The clinical consequences of cholesterol crystal embolism are variable. Embolization may be completely asymptomatic and the diagnosis made at renal biopsy, or cause an ischemic digit or a multisystem disease that mimics systemic vasculitis. The distribution of end-organ damage depends on the location of the original atherosclerotic plaques.

15.2.1 Clinical Features

Clinically significant renal involvement occurs in around 50 % of patients [1], the onset of renal disease after the triggering event may be immediate but can be more insidious with a delay of weeks or months. There may be acute renal impairment following massive embolization, alternatively there may be a gradual deterioration in renal function due to crystal embolic showers, or an ischemic nephropathy.

Cutaneous manifestations are typically ischemic digits, particularly the toes from abdominal atheroma emboli, or a livedo reticularis appearance typically affecting the legs. Limb ischemia usually presents as sudden onset of a small, cool, cyanotic and painful area of the foot (usually the toe). The lesions are tender to touch and may progress to ulceration, digital infarction, and gangrene. The peripheral pulses are usually well-preserved despite the digital cyanosis (Fig. 15.1). Other common features include abdominal pain, central nervous system involvement, fever, and weight loss.

15.2.2 Laboratory Features

Laboratory investigations are often nonspecific including uremia, thrombocytopenia, eosinophilia, elevated ESR, hypocomplementemia and disseminated intravascular coagulation. ANCA is not usually detected in the serum. Diagnosis is based on the clinical features with a typical history, supported

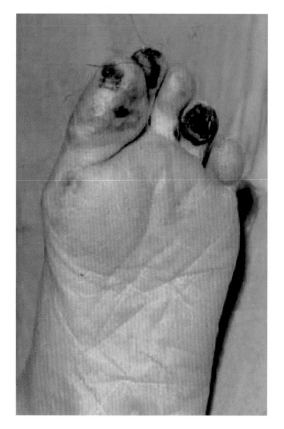

FIGURE 15.1 Ischemic digits in cholesterol embolism

by histological demonstration of the typical cholesterol clefts or cholesterol emboli in vessels (Fig. 15.2).

15.2.3   Treatment

Treatment is aimed at halting the progression of tissue ischemia and prevention of further embolization. Anticoagulation should be avoided as this may exacerbate embolization. Antiplatelet therapy is unsuccessful. Modification of traditional risk factors for atherosclerosis such as smoking, hypertension and hypercholsterolaemia is essential.

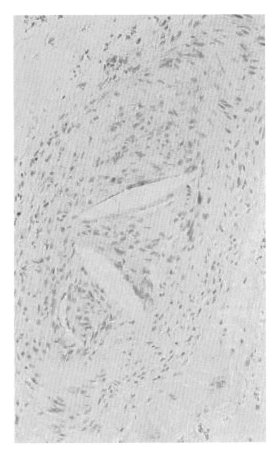

FIGURE 15.2 Skin biopsy from a patient with cholesterol embolism showing typical cleft due to cholesterol emboli. The cholesterol has dissolved during processing leaving the cleft

15.3   Calciphylaxis

Calciphylaxis is rare, but potentially fatal. It occurs in patients with chronic renal failure with secondary hyperparathyroidism. Disturbance of calcium and phosphate metabolism results in painful necrosis of skin, subcutaneous tissue, and acral gangrene. Appearance of the lesions is distinctive but the pathogenesis remains uncertain. Correction of hyperphosphatemia or occasionally hypercalcemia is vital, and parathyroidectomy may be of benefit [3].

15.4   Cardiac Myxoma

Cardiac myxomata are rare benign tumors most commonly found in 90 % of cases in the left atrium.

15.4.1   Clinical Features

Constitutional symptoms and systemic embolization may lead to an erroneous diagnosis of vasculitis [4].

Systemic manifestations are seen in 90 % of cases including: fever, weight loss, Raynaud's phenomenon, clubbing, elevated acute phase proteins, and hypergammaglobulinemia. Systemic embolization occurs in 40 %; emboli may be large enough to occlude the aortic bifurcation, and smaller emboli may remain viable and invade the vessel wall resulting in aneurysm formation that mimics PAN. The diagnosis is made by echocardiography, which should be performed in all cases of suspected systemic vasculitis.

15.4.2   Treatment

Treatment is by surgical resection of the primary tumor and any emboli.

15.5   Infective Endocarditis

Infective endocarditis is associated with both true vasculitis and embolic phenomenon. True vasculitic lesions are caused either by an immune complex vasculitis, or mycotic aneurysm formation by septic emboli where there is a direct invasion of the vessel wall. Petechiae, strokes, splenic infarcts, and glomerulonephritis are the most extracardiac common features. There is an immunology response with elevation of acute phase proteins, hypergammaglobulinemia, and autoantibody formation. The diagnosis is made by blood culture and echocardiography.

15.6   Fibromuscular Dysplasia

Fibromuscular dysplasia is a vascular disease that affects small to medium arteries. It is a noninflammatory, nonatherosclerotic condition that occurs in young adults and is four times more common in women than men. Renal artery involvement occurs in 60–75 %, cervicocranial arteries in 25–30 %, visceral arteries in 9 %, and peripheral arteries in 5 % of cases [5]. Classification is dependent on the dominant arterial wall layer involved: intimal, medial, and adventitial. The etiology is unknown, but there is a strong genetic component. Clinical manifestations reflect the arterial tree involved with renovascular hypertension, renal infarction, dissection, transient ischemic attacks, and stroke. The diagnosis is made on the typical digital subtraction angiographic appearances with the classic "string of beads appearance." Fibromuscular dysplasia, in particular, diffuse intimal disease can occasionally be difficult to distinguish from vasculitis especially, Takayasu arteritis. There should not however be evidence of an acute phase response. Symptomatic stenotic lesions are treated by percutaneous transluminal angioplasty or bypass grafting, together with antiplatelet drugs. Digital subtraction angiography is the gold standard test, but the diagnosis can be made using magnetic resonance angiography or CT angiography. Doppler ultrasound may show aneurysm but needs to be confirmed with angiography [6].

15.7   Chronic Ergotism

Epidemic ergotism occurs after ingestion of grain contaminated with ergot (*Claviceps purpurea*) [7]. Since medieval times, epidemics have been described in which painful gangrene of the peripheries occurred with loss of extremities.

Critical mesenteric ischemia can occur. Chronic ergotism can occur following long-term use of ergotamine tartrate to treat migraine. Peripheral, carotid, coronary, and visceral ischemia may develop. The contrast angiographic appearances may simulate vasculitis with irregular, long or short segmental stenosis. The diagnosis is dependent on a history of ergot consumption. The lesions may not be fully reversible on withdrawal of ergot.

15.8   Köhlmeier–Degos Disease

Köhlmeier–Degos disease (malignant atrophic papulosis) is a rare and lethal condition, which involves skin, gut, and the nervous system. The typical skin lesions begin as erythematosus, pink or red papules (2–15 mm diameter), which evolve into circular porcelain white scars with an atrophic depressed center. The arterial lesion is luminal stenosis or occlusion due to intimal proliferation and consequent thrombosis presentation is with acute abdominal pain leading to bowel infarction, fever, acute phase response in association with the skin lesion. The multisystem nature of Köhlmeier–Degos disease mimics a vasculitis. The diagnosis is made on biopsy. There is no specific therapy. The usual cause of death is intestinal perforation [8].

15.9   Cryofibrinogenemia

Cryofibrinogenemia occurs when a cryoprecipitate occurs in plasma, which has been anticoagulated with oxalate, citrate or edetic acid. The cryoprecipitate is a complex, which includes a number of plasma proteins including fibrin, fibrinogen, and fibrin split products. The cryofibrinogen is consumed in the clotting process and therefore unlike a cryoglobulin does not precipitate in cooled serum. In many cases (88 %) there is an associated cryoglobulin. Cryofibrinogenemia may be asymptomatic but can present with purpura (47 %), skin necrosis (37 %), ulcers, gangrene, arthralgias (32 %), glomerulonephritis, or a leukocytoclastic

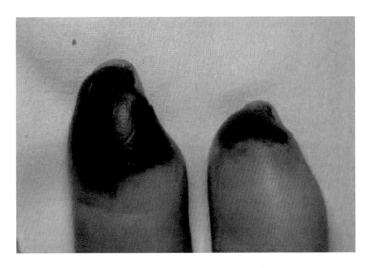

FIGURE 15.3 Ischemic digits in cryofibrinogenemia

vasculitis [9], and thus mimic a systemic vasculitis (Fig. 15.3). Cryofibrinogenemia may be primary or secondary to malignancy, infection, or a connective tissue disease. Treatment is by cold avoidance and treatment of the underlying condition, combined with immunosuppression, plasmapheresis and antithrombotic drugs.

15.10   Radiation Vasculopathy

Radiation has been known to cause vascular injury since the early 1900s. Acute vascular injury occurs within hours of large doses of radiation and presents with hypotension, shock, and death. Chronic radiation vasculopathy present with (i) internal injury and mural thrombosis occurring within 5 years; (ii) progressive sclerosis of arterioles and arteries occurring within 10 years and which can lead to luminal occlusion; and (iii) accelerated atherosclerosis with a latency of 20 years. The endothelial cell is the most radiation sensitive part of the vascular system.

Clinically, the manifestations depend on the organs included in the field of radiation, and the dose, and type of radiation used. Features include arterial stenosis and occlusion, rupture and aneurysms formation. The angiographic appearance is similar to those seen on atherosclerosis. Radiation vasculopathy can be distinguished from systemic vasculitis by the history of irradiation and the lack of an acute phase response.

15.11   Cocaine Abuse

Intranasal cocaine use as a recreational drug can lead to destructive midline lesions of the nose [10]. These lesions can be very difficult to distinguish from those seen in granulomatosis with polyangiitis (Wegener's) as they can present with midline facial pain, epistaxis and a systemic illness. Septal perforation with necrosis of sinus mucosa can occur and ANCA may be present in the serum. The ANCA pattern may be atypical. A very careful history is required to establish cocaine use as the patient may initially deny its use. Treatment with immunosuppressive therapy may not be needed if cocaine is withdrawn. Surgical repair of the nasal defect may be difficult.

15.12   Scurvy

Privational vitamin C deficiency is a rare diagnosis in the developed world. Scurvy can be readily precipitated by a vitamin C deficient diet (e.g., a diet devoid of fruit and vegetables), as humans cannot synthesize vitamin C. Diagnosis of scurvy is generally based on clinical features and dietary history, as well as rapid resolution of signs and symptoms after vitamin C supplementation.

The common symptoms of scurvy include bruising, arthralgias, petechiae, or joint swelling. Nonspecific pedal edema, bruising, and gingival involvement are also quite common. Dermatological features include broken or coiled hairs with perifollicular hemorrhages and hyperkeratosis. Musculoskeletal features include painful hemarthrosis, and subperiosteal hemorrhage.

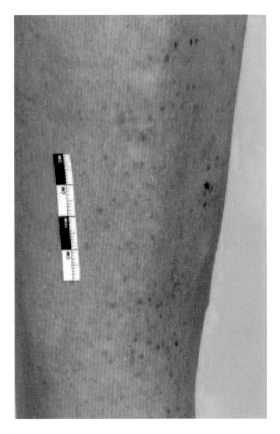

FIGURE 15.4 Pseudovasculitic rash occurring in a patient with privational scurvy

The rash can be mistaken for a systemic vasculitis (Fig. 15.4) [11], however a skin biopsy should enable the diagnosis to be made as features of vasculitis will be absent and there will be evidence of perifollicular hemorrhage.

15.13   Sweet's Syndrome

Sweet's syndrome (acute febrile neutrophilic dermatosis) is an inflammatory neutrophil dermatosis. The infiltrate consists of mature polymorphonuclear leucocytes located in the

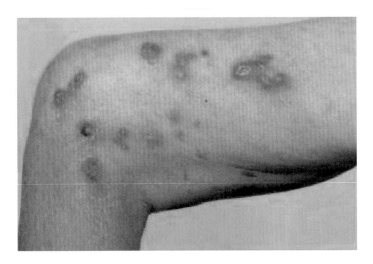

FIGURE 15.5 Sweet's syndrome

dermis. The condition is characterized by pyrexia, elevation of white cell count, painful erythematosus cutaneous lesions (Fig. 15.5) [12]. Sweet's syndrome can be associated with drug and malignancy. The cutaneous lesions in association with a systemic illness may be mistaken for vasculitis but the diagnosis is made on biopsy. Treatment is with glucocorticoids.

Key Points
- The manifestations of vasculitis are protean and a number of conditions may mimic vasculitis.
- A high index of suspicion must be maintained for mimics.
- Cholesterol embolism and infective endocarditis are the two most typical mimics.

References

1. Scolari F, Tardanico R, Pola A, et al. Cholesterol crystal embolism: a recognizable cause of renal disease. Am J Kidney Dis. 2000;36:1089–99.

2. Kronzon I, Saric M. Cholesterol embolism syndrome. Circulation. 2010;122:631–41.
3. Mathur RV, Shortland JR, el-Nahas AM. Calciphylaxis. Postgrad Med J. 2001;77:557–61.
4. Boussen K, et al. Embolisation of cardiac myxoma masquerading as polyarteritis nodosa. J Rheumatol. 1991;18:283–5.
5. Begelman SM, Olin JW. Fibromuscular dysplasia. Curr Opin Rheumatol. 2000;12:41–7.
6. Pluoin P-F, Perdu J, Batide-Alanore AL, Boutouyrie P, Gimenez-Roqueplo A-P, Jeunemaitre X. Fibromuscular dysplasia. Orphanet J Rare Dis. 2007;2:28–36.
7. Christopoulos S, Szilagyi A, Kahn SR. Saint Anthony's fire. Lancet. 2001;358:1694.
8. Scheinfeld N. Malignant atrophic papulosis. Clin Exp Dermatol. 2007;32:483–7.
9. Michaud M, Pourrat J. Cryofibrinogenaemia. J Clin Rheumatol. 2012;19:142–8.
10. Rachapalli S, Kiely P. Cocaine-induced midline destructive lesions mimicking ENT-limited Wegener's granulomatosis. Scand J Rheumatol. 2008;37:477–80.
11. Sithamparanathan K, Dubey S, Garber S, Watts R. Scurvy: MRI appearances. Rheumatology. 2008;47:1109.
12. Chen PR. Neutrophilic dermatoses: a review of current treatment options. Am J Clin Dermatol. 2009;10:301–12.

Chapter 16
Secondary Vasculitis

16.1 Introduction

Vasculitis often occurs as a primary event (*de novo*), but can occur on the background of a number of other diseases; in particular, it is associated with certain infections, drugs, and connective tissue diseases such as rheumatoid arthritis and SLE. It can also occur in association with some malignancies.

16.2 Definition

Secondary vasculitis describes systemic vasculitis occurring on the background of other diseases or known infections/or associated with drug treatment.

16.3 Epidemiology

There is little data on the incidence of secondary vasculitis. Systemic vasculitis complicating rheumatoid arthritis has become much less frequent over the last two decades [1], but there is little evidence of any major change in association with other trigger factors.

R.A. Watts et al., *Vasculitis in Clinical Practice*,
DOI 10.1007/978-3-319-14871-7_16,
© Springer International Publishing AG, Cham 2015

16.4   Etiology

Some drugs originally associated with vasculitis, particularly hydralazine and penicillamine, are now used much less frequently. There are, however, reports of EGPA associated with leukotriene inhibitors and the commonest cause of ANCA-associated vasculitis secondary to drug treatment is propylthiouracil.

16.5   Infection and Vasculitis

The association between infection and vasculitis has been recognized for many years and a number of different organisms identified (see Table 16.1).

TABLE 16.1 Infection and vasculitis

Vessel involved		Infection
Large arteries	Bacterial	Staphylococcus, Salmonella, mycobacteria, Streptococcus
	Spirochaetal	Treponema pallidum
	Fungal	coccidioidomycosis
Medium arteries	Bacterial	Group A Streptoccus, mycobacteria
	Viral	HBV, HCV, HIV, parvovirus B19
Small vessels and medium arteries	Bacterial	Streptococcus
	Viral	HBV, HCV, HIV, CMV
	Bacterial	Staphylococcus, Salmonella, mycobacteria, Streptococcus, Yersinia, Neisseria, Rickettsiae
Small vessel (leukocytoclastic)	Viral	HIV, CMV, herpes zoster, parvovirus B19, HBV, HCV

Adapted from Somer and Finegold [2]
CMV cytomegalovirus', *HBV* hepatitis B virus, *HCV* hepatitis C virus, *HIV* human immunodeficiency virus

The most widely publicized association is between hepatitis B (HBV) and polyarteritis nodosa. This association was first described over 40 years ago and the highest reported incidence of PAN was 77 per million in an area endemic for HBV infection. In France, falling HBV infection rate has correlated with a significant decrease in HBV-associated PAN [3]. In our population in Norwich we find this to be very rare. The common clinical features are very similar to classic PAN with mononeuritis multiplex (83.5 %), GI involvement (57 %), renal tract (38 %), skin (31 %), and hypertension (31 %) [3]. HBV-associated PAN usually develops within 12 months of infection and hepatitis is often quite mild. Angiography will show typical microaneurysms and/or stenosis in the celiac axis and renal blood vessels. ANCA are not associated with HBV vasculitis.

Treatment for HBV-associated vasculitis is with a combination of antiviral agents, together with plasma exchange (see Table 16.2).

Hepatitis C is also associated with vasculitis, but almost always with cryoglobulinemia and cryoglobulinemic vasculitis (see Chap. 14). Other viruses associated with vasculitis are as shown in Table 16.2.

Direct invasion of blood vessel wall by pyogenic organisms (most often staphylococcus and streptococcus) can also cause vasculitis. It is often associated with a predisposing condition such as diabetes mellitus and may occur at a site of previous damage by atheroma or surgery.

Large artery involvement is rare, but when it occurs, the usual process is by the formation of mycotic aneurysms. This is most commonly associated with streptococcus pneumonii and salmonella, although often in association with underlying/predisposing conditions such as diabetes or intravenous drug use.

There are descriptions of vasculitis also associated with mycobacteria, spirochetes (*Treponema pallidum* associated with aortitis), and rickettsia, usually presenting with an extensive maculopapular rash in patients with rocky mountain spotted fever and also fungal infections – mainly associated with immunocompromised patients involving both CNS and large arteries (mycotic aneurysm formation).

TABLE 16.2 Major viruses associated with vasculitis and their treatment

Virus	Type of vasculitis	Standard therapy
HBV	PAN	Short CS, PE, Lamivudine
HCV	Cryoglobulinemic vasculitis	Short CS, IFNx, and ribavirin ± PE
HIV	PAN large/medium/small vessel vasculitis Cerebral vasculitis	Short CS with ARV ± PE
Parvovirus	PAN	CS
B19	"HSP"-like	CS and/or Mg
Varicella zoster	Retinitis meningoencephalomyelitis	Aciclovir ± CS
CMV	Retinitis Colitis PAN	Valganciclovir, ganciclovir or foscarnet

Adapted from Pagnoux et al. [4]
ARV anti-retroviral drugs, *CMV* cytomegalovirus, *CS* glucococorticoid, *HBV* hepatitis B virus, *HCV* hepatitis C virus. *HIV* human immunodeficiency virus, *HSP* Henoch–Schönlein purpura (now called IgA vasculitis), *PAN* polyarteritis nodosa, *PE* plasma exchange

16.6   Vasculitis and Malignancy

Acute vasculitis may be the presenting feature of a variety of malignancies (Table 16.3).

This is relatively infrequent, with one review suggesting one in a thousand patients with malignancy developing vasculitis. Half the cases of cancer and vasculitis occurred within the first 12 months after the malignancy. Vasculitis is classically a cutaneous leukocytoclastic vasculitis, but occasionally, malignancy is associated with giant-cell arteritis, polyarteritis nodosa, and even GPA. Malignancy also appears to be associated with certain types of vasculitis. For example, malignancy was found in up to 5 % of patients

TABLE 16.3 Pattern of vasculitis occurring in association with malignancy

Malignancy developing in patients with a diagnosis of primary systemic vasculitis	Malignancies associated with subsequent development of vasculitis	Types of vasculitis associated with malignancy
Renal Cell carcinoma	Myelodysplasia lymphoma	GPA
Colon adenocarcinoma	Hairy cell leukemia	Polyarteritis nodosa
Skin	Myeloma	MPA
Leukemia		IgA vasculitis
Lymphoma		Cutaneous leukocytoclastic vasculitis
Bladder carcinoma[a]		

[a]Cyclophosphamide treatment associated

with GPA compared to 3 % of patients with rheumatoid arthritis. The commonest association appears to be between renal cell carcinoma and GPA [5]. Other cancers appear to occur in the same numbers as might be expected in a normal population, but there are reports describing colon cancer in association with IgA vasculitis and microscopic polyangiitis.

The most recent description of malignancy was in the WEGT study [6], which described an increased frequency of solid malignancies in patients with GPA treated with etanercept. Whether this was the result of treatment is uncertain. This study showed an association with colon cancer, cholangiocarcinoma, breast cancer, and renal cell carcinoma.

IgA vasculitis has also been described in association with malignancy, but there does not appear to be any risk other than that seen in other types of vasculitis or autoimmune disease.

Vasculitis associated with lymphoproliferative disease disorders is usually localized to the skin and again is rare (2.3 % in one series) [7]. Vasculitis has also been described in association with myelodysplastic syndrome in up to 10 % of cases. Hairy cell leukemia is a rare lymphoproliferative disease, which can present in a systemic way similar to polyarteritis nodosa, as well as cutaneous leukocytoclastic vasculitis. The histology shows direct infiltration of the vessel wall by malignant cells in some cases. There may be an interval of several years between the vasculitis and the hairy cell leukemia.

Finally, vasculitis may also mimic malignancy, and the differentiation between lymphoma and GPA, for example, in the upper airways can be extremely difficult.

The risk of bladder cancer developing in patients given long-term oral cyclophosphomide goes on for many years [8]. One study showed a 31 fold increased risk of bladder cancer in patients with GPA receiving treatment. This risk appears to be associated with total dose exposure and the trend is now, therefore, to use shorter courses of treatment and intermittent treatment where there appears to be lower risk. Lymphoma and skin malignancy and leukemias may also be increased as a consequence of immunosuppressive therapy.

16.7   Drug-Induced Vasculitis

A very wide range of drugs, vaccines, and desensitization procedures have been reported in association with vasculitis. Many are isolated case reports and it is often difficult to conclusively prove any causal relation. The most recent best described associations have been with propylthiouracil and the leukotriene antagonists [9, 10]. Propylthiouracil is particularly associated with ANCA-associated vasculitis. The link between leukotriene antagonists, which have been used to treat asthma, and the onset of EGPA has been the subject of much discussion. Current thinking is that use of leukotriene antagonists allows EGPA to become manifest as steroids are withdrawn, rather than there be a causal link. Most vasculitis

associated with drugs is small vessel vasculitis and occasionally medium vessel vasculitis, though large vessel vasculitis is
very rare.

Clinical features depend on the presentation. With the
leukotriene antagonists, they are all typical features of
EGPA. In other drug-induced vasculitis, the commonest
involvement is in the skin with purpura, which may be palpable and the lesions may scar. Histology shows a leukocytoclastic vasculitis. Other non-specific laboratory findings
include leukocytosis, hypocomplementemia, and a raised
acute phase response. Eosinophilia is not uncommon, but
when very high levels of peripheral blood eosinophils are
seen, it is usually indicative of the evolution to EGPA (see
above).

The ANCA associated with propylthiouracil is usually of
antimyeloperoxidase (MPO) specificity, and although rare, it
is important to consider this drug in all patients presenting
with an ANCA-associated vasculitis.

16.8   Systemic Rheumatoid Vasculitis

Vasculitis has been known to be associated with rheumatoid
arthritis for many years. Recent studies have suggested that
this complication is becoming increasingly rare, falling from
approximately 10 per million in the 1970s and 80s to less than
3 per million by the 1990s and the incidence appears to have
been relatively stable since then [1]. Whether this is due to
improved treatment is uncertain. This finding has been
described in detail in the UK and North America.

Classic patients who develop rheumatoid vasculitis have
seropositive disease, often with other extra articular manifestations such as nodules and pulmonary fibrosis. The commonest findings are nailfold or nail bed infarcts (Fig. 16.1).
A similar vasculitis to that seen in the ANCA-associated
vasculitis is also well described. Treatment of systemic rheumatoid vasculitis is similar to that for ANCA-associated vasculitis with cyclophosphomide and steroids [11]. The prognosis

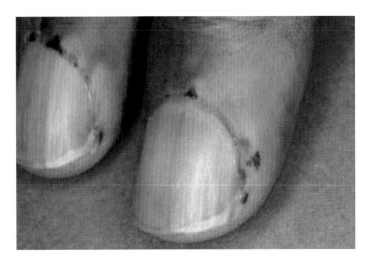

FIGURE 16.1 Nailfold vasculitis in a patient with rheumatoid arthritis

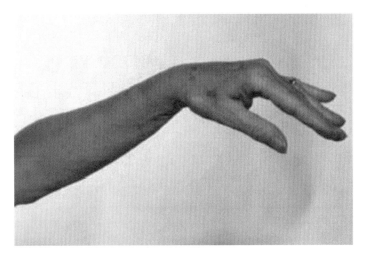

FIGURE 16.2 Mononeuritis multiplex causing a wrist drop in a patient with systemic rheumatoid vasculitis

in the past has been poor, particularly in patients who have neuropathy (Fig. 16.2), peripheral gangrene, and/or histological evidence of an arteritis as opposed to small vessel leukocytoclastic vasculitis. A recent review suggests that although the frequency of the disease has dramatically fallen the prognosis in the modern era has not improved [1].

The laboratory features associated with systemic rheumatoid vasculitis are similar to those of ANCA-associated vasculitis, except these patients are ANCA negative. This means that they have evidence of an acute phase response, sometimes anemia, leukocytosis, and abnormal liver function tests usually associated with inflammation, i.e., raised gamma-glutamyl transferase and alkaline phosphatase. Some patients have hypocomplementemia, particularly low C4, and about 50 % of patients are ANA positive. It is one of the few occasions when it is worth repeating the rheumatoid factor titer, which is often at very high levels, and occasionally, patients have cryoglobulinemia which is a mixed cryoglobulinemia including rheumatoid factor. Research studies have shown association with IgA and IgG rheumatoid factor, but these are not routinely measured in clinical practice.

When nailfold or digital infarcts are the only clinical manifestation of vasculitis, i.e., there is no evidence of systemic illness and no extraarticular disease such as pericarditis, etc., then the natural history is relatively benign. Only a small percentage of patients develop systemic features during follow-up and this is usually relatively early on, within 3–6 months.

Vasculitis has very rarely been described as the presenting feature of rheumatoid arthritis. The clinical feature in reported cases has been a peripheral neuropathy.

16.9 Systemic Lupus Erythematosus

Cutaneous vasculitis is a very common feature of SLE and biopsy of many of the cutaneous manifestations can include small vessel vasculitis. Involvement of arterioles arteries, mimicking the ANCA-associated vasculitis, is extremely rare but associated with a particularly poor prognosis. Patients have typical autoantibodies associated with lupus including ANA, DNA binding, hypocomplementemia, and sometimes Ro and La antibodies (see below).

Clinical features sometimes associated with systemic vasculitis and lupus include peripheral neuropathy, particularly mononeuritis multiplex. Rapidly progressive glomerulonephritis may also sometimes be associated with systemic vasculitis. Treatment of lupus associated vasculitis is similar to that for the ANCA associated vasculitides (see Chap. 4).

16.10   Sjögren's Syndrome

A cutaneous leukocytoclastic vasculitis is not an infrequent complication of primary Sjögren's syndrome. It is associated particularly with those who are seropositive for Ro and La antibodies. Although cutaneous vasculitis is the commonest feature (Fig. 16.3), patients occasionally develop a focal segmental necrotizing glomerulonephritis similar to that seen in lupus and in the ANCA associated vasculitides. Treatment is as for the ANCA-associated vasculitis and systemic vasculitis complicating SLE.

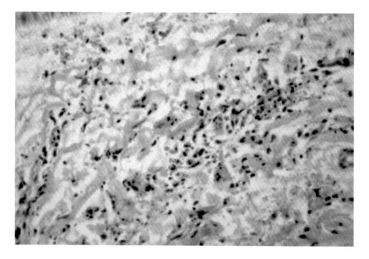

Figure 16.3 Cutaneous vasculitis in a patient with Sjögren's syndrome

16.11   Spondyloarthopathies

Unlike the other connective tissue diseases, the commonest form of vascular involvement in ankylosing spondylitis is an aortitis particularly affecting the aortic root and ascending aorta. Very occasional distal aortitis can occur. Inflammation of the aortic root can be associated with aortic regurgitation and the evidence for this development increases with the duration of ankylosing spondylitis and may be as high as 10 % at 30 years [12]. The aortitis is investigated by echocardiography which shows thickening of the aortic leaflets. Histology shows lymphocytic infiltration possibly with fibrosis in the aortic wall and the aortic roots. There is no data as to the appropriate treatment of the aortitis associated which ankylosing spondylitis, but anecdotal reports that immunosuppressive drugs should be used if there is evidence of active inflammation and that surgery is particularly risky if the inflammation is not controlled.

Key Points
- Systemic rheumatoid vasculitis is becoming less common.
- Infection should be considered in the differential diagnosis of any patient presenting with systemic rheumatoid vasculitis.
- Drug-induced vasculitis is quite common and should always be considered in patients presenting predominately cutaneous involvement.

References

1. Ntatsaki E, Mooney J, Scott DGI, Watts RA. Systemic Rheumatoid Vasculitis in the era of modern immunosuppressive therapy. Rheumatology (Oxford). 2014;53(1):145–52.
2. Somer T, Finegold SM. Vasculitis associated with infections, immunization, and antimicrobial drugs. Clin Infect Dis. 1995;20:1010–36.

3. Guillevin L, Mahr A, Callard P, et al. Hepatitis B virus associated polyarteritis nodosa. Clinical characteristics, outcome and impact of treatment in 115 patients. Medicine (Baltimore). 2005;84:313–22.
4. Pagnoux C, Cohen P, Guillevin L. Vasculitis secondary to infections. Clin Exp Rheumatol. 2006;24 Suppl 2:S71–81.
5. Tatsis E, Reinhold-Keller E, Steindorf K, Feller AC, Gross WL. Wegener's granulomatosis associated with renal cell carcinoma. Arthritis Rheum. 1999;42:751–6.
6. Stone JH, Holbrook JT, Marriott MA, et al. Solid malignancies among patients in the Wegener's Granulomatosis Etanercept Trial. Arthritis Rheum. 2006;54:1608–18.
7. Hamidou MA, Derenne S, Audrain MA, Berthelot JM, Boumalassa A, Grolleau JY. Prevalence of rheumatic manifestations and antineutrophil cytoplasmic antibodies in haematological malignancies. A prospective study. Rheumatology (Oxford). 2000;39:417–20.
8. Knight A, Askling J, Granath F, Sparen P, Ekbom A. Urinary bladder cancer in Wegener's granulomatosis: risks and relation to cyclophosphamide. Ann Rheum Dis. 2004;63(10):1307–11.
9. Choi HK, Merkel PA, Walker AM, Niles JL. Drug-associated antineutrophil cytoplasmic antibody-positive vasculitis: prevalence among patients with high titers of antimyeloperoxidase antibodies. Arthritis Rheum. 2000;43:405–13.
10. Wechsler ME, Finn D, Gunawardena D, et al. Churg–Strauss syndrome in patients receiving montelukast as treatment for asthma. Chest. 2000;117:708–13.
11. Scott DG, Bacon PA. Intravenous cyclophosphamide plus methylprednisolone in treatment of systemic rheumatoid vasculitis. Am J Med. 1984;76:377–84.
12. Townend JN, Emery P, Davies MK, Littler WA. Acute aortitis and aortic incompetence due to systemic rheumatological disorders. Int J Cardiol. 1991;33:253–8.

Chapter 17
Primary Angiitis of the Central Nervous System Vasculitis

17.1 Introduction

Vasculitis affecting the central nervous system is one of the rarest forms of vasculitis, which combined with the complexity of investigation of CNS function has made the establishment of clear diagnostic criteria and treatment regimens very difficult.

In broad terms, CNS vasculitis can be broken down into primary and secondary forms.

17.2 Definition and Classification

Primary angiitis of the central nervous system (PACNS) occurs when the disease process is confined to the brain, spinal cord, and overlying leptomeninges. Secondary CNS vasculitis can occur in any condition where there is vascular inflammation such as systemic vasculitis, infections, and lymphoproliferative disease.

There are no validated criteria for the diagnosis of PACNS. Classification is usually based on; (i) a history of acquired unexplained neurological deficit; (ii) high probability angiographic or histopathological evidence of angiitis in the CNS; (iii) no evidence of systemic vasculitis or other condition to which the angiographic appearance could be attributed [1]. PACNS once diagnosed is categorized into one of

R.A. Watts et al., *Vasculitis in Clinical Practice*,
DOI 10.1007/978-3-319-14871-7_17,
© Springer International Publishing AG, Cham 2015

the recognized subsets or clinical variants such as granuloma-tous angiitis, benign angiopathy, and atypical. CNS angiitis may be associated with varicella zoster, sarcoid, or amyloido-sis [2]. These subsets appear to have varyingly important prognostic and therapeutic implications.

17.3   Epidemiology

There is a reported female predominance, and no age-group is known to be particularly prone to developing the condition. The annual incidence is 2.4/million in Olmsted County (USA).

17.4   Etiology

The etiology of PACNS is unknown. Secondary forms are associated with herpes zoster infection, sarcoid, and amyloidosis.

17.5   Clinical Features

17.5.1   Systemic

Systemic features normally associated with systemic vasculi-tis such as fever and weight loss are relatively uncommon.

17.5.2   Neurological

The most common clinical manifestations are headache and behavioral/mental changes. The rate of onset of these symptoms can vary from weeks to months. Focal neuro-logical signs are often the main presenting symptom, com-monly, aphasia, hemiparesis, or seizures. Visual defects occur in approximately 21 % and decreased visual acuity in 11 %.

17.6   Laboratory Features

Blood-based investigations are largely unhelpful in the diagnosis of primary CNS vasculitis. They are however important to exclude secondary CNS vasculitis; hence, autoantibody screening, clinical chemistry, and microbiological tests should be performed. Investigations are important to establish the extent of organ involvement.

FBC is typically normal. The acute phase response (ESR and CRP) is infrequently elevated. ANCA, ANA, RF, anticardiolipin antibodies, complement, and cryoglobulins are normal or negative.

17.6.1   Cerebrospinal Fluid

Abnormalities in the CSF are found in 88 % of patients. The white cell count is typically elevated with an increase in total protein. The white count is rarely over 250 cell/mm^3 and the protein >500 mg%. Red blood cells are found in 79 %.

17.6.2   Imaging

Neuroimaging studies are vital in the diagnostic workup. Cerebral MRI is abnormal in 97 % patients. The most common lesion is cerebral infarction seen in half of patients, and the majority of patients have multiple infarctions, often bilateral and involving the cortex and subcortex. Intracranial hemorrhage is unusual (<10 %). Gadolinium-enhancing lesions may be seen in one-third of patients. Enhancement of the leptomeninges may be seen and can be used to guide biopsy. Typically, on cerebral angiography, changes are found in multiple vessels, usually bilateral. Involvement of small vessels is more common than large vessels. The angiogram may be normal in up to 40 % of patients and the findings nonspecific in a further 20 %.

17.6.3   Pathology

A biopsy of both leptomeninges and brain is necessary to make a definitive diagnosis and is positive in 75 % of patients. Histology may show a granulomatous vasculitis with or without acute necrosis. A lymphocytic pattern may be seen. The major role of biopsy is to exclude other forms of vascular inflammation, malignancy, and infection.

17.6.4   Electroencephalography

There are no specific features seen on electroencephalography; possible findings include dysrhythmias, epileptogenic changes, and delta waves.

17.7   Diagnosis

The diagnosis of CNS angiitis is most commonly considered in a patient with an unexplained neurological event and CSF findings consistent with chronic meningitis.

The differential diagnosis is from malignancy, infection, sarcoid, and amyloidosis. The recent description of a syndrome of reversible cerebral vasoconstriction should also be considered – this is characterized clinically by recurrent thunderclap headache with or without neurological deficit and normal CSF analysis findings and angiographically by reversible diffuse segmental vasospasm of intracranial vessels [3].

The diagnosis is usually made on a combination of MRI, angiography, CSF, and biopsy findings.

17.8   Assessment of Disease Activity

Assessment of disease activity is based largely on the patient's clinical condition and response to treatment. Inflammatory markers are not a reliable guide to disease activity and the neuroimaging described has not been validated for disease monitoring.

17.9   Treatment

There are no controlled trials to guide therapy. Induction therapy involves high-dose corticosteroids, 1 mg/kg up to maximum 60 mg with a rapid tapering down to 10 mg at 6 months. In severe cases i.v. methylprednisolone is indicated. In patients with a poor prognostic outcome consider using i.v. cyclophosphamide. Maintenance therapy is with oral corticosteroids with a tapering dose of prednisolone. The majority of patients require treatment for less than 18 months. A relapse in disease is treated with an increase in prednisolone dosage and the introduction of other immunosuppressive agents such as cyclophosphamide or azathioprine. Refractory disease may require treatment with agents such as mycophenolate mofetil or biological agents, but currently, there is little evidence to support their use.

17.10   Prognosis

PACNS is associated with increased mortality compared with the general population. Poor prognosis is associated with the following at presentation: neurological deficit, cerebral infarction, and large vessel involvement.

Cerebral infarction is a frequent cause of death. Relapse has been shown to occur in approximately one quarter of patients followed for 13 months.

Key Points
- Vasculitis limited to the brain, spinal cord, and overlying leptomeninges.
- Confirmed by either biopsy of tissues within the central nervous system or cerebral angiography.
- Confirmed only after meticulous exclusion of all conditions capable of producing vasculitis within the nervous system.

References

1. Calabrese H, Mallek JA. Primary angiitis of the central nervous system: report of 8 new cases, review of the literature, and proposal for diagnostic criteria. Medicine (Baltimore). 1988; 67:20–39.
2. Salvarani C, Brown RD, Calamia KT, et al. Primary central nervous system vasculitis: analysis of 101 patients. Annal Neurol. 2007;62:442–51.
3. Hammad TA, Hajj-Ali RA. Primary angiitis of the central nervous system and reversible cerebral vasoconstriction syndrome. Curr Atheroscler Rep. 2013;15(8):346.

Chapter 18
Relapsing Polychondritis

18.1 Introduction

Relapsing polychondritis (RP) is a rare condition characterized by inflammation and destruction of cartilage.

18.2 Definition and Classification

There are no validated diagnostic criteria, however a diagnosis of RP should be considered if at least three of the features
given in Table 18.1 are present, or one of the clinical features
with a biopsy confirmation or chondritis at two or more loca-
tions which responds to treatment with steroids and/or dapsone [1].

18.3 Epidemiology

The incidence of RP has been estimated to be 3.5/million in
Rochester County, USA. Males and females are affected
equally, and the peak age of onset is 50 years.

Relapsing polychondritis is more common around the
Mediterranean littoral, the Silk Route and Japan, but has
been described in every ethnic group.

R.A. Watts et al., *Vasculitis in Clinical Practice*,
DOI 10.1007/978-3-319-14871-7_18,
© Springer International Publishing AG, Cham 2015

TABLE 18.1 Characteristic features of RP

Recurrent chondritis of both auricles
Non-erosive seronegative inflammatory polyarthritis
Nasal chondritis
Inflammation of ocular structures (conjunctivitis, keratitis, scleritis, episcleritis, uveitis)
Chondritis of the respiratory tract involving laryngeal and/or tracheal cartilage
Cochlear and/or vestibular damage causing sensorineural hearing loss, tinnitus and/or vertigo

18.4   Etiology

The etiology is unknown, but like many autoimmune conditions, is generally believed to result from an environmental trigger interacting with a genetically predisposed host. Familial cases are rare. There is an association with HLA-DR4. No infectious triggers have been identified. There is frequently a co-existent autoimmune disease. Antibodies to type II collagen are found.

18.5   Clinical Features

18.5.1   Systemic

The initial symptoms may be nonspecific with fever, weight loss and fatigue.

18.5.2   Cartilage Inflammation

Auricular inflammation is present in almost all patients (85 %) (Fig. 18.1). This involves the cartilaginous part of the pinna and spares the noncartilaginous lobe. The pinna becomes red,

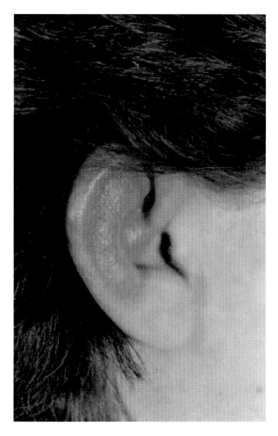

FIGURE 18.1 Auricular inflammation in a patient with relapsing polychondritis (RP)

painful, swollen, and these inflammatory episodes last a few days or weeks. Following recurrent inflammation, the pinna becomes floppy and loses its rigidity. There may be inflammation of the middle ear and audiovestibular structures.

Nasal chondritis occurs in 50 % of cases, presenting with pain, erythema, swelling, and stuffiness. The cartilage within the nasal bridge is destroyed and collapses, leading to a saddle nose deformity (Fig. 18.2).

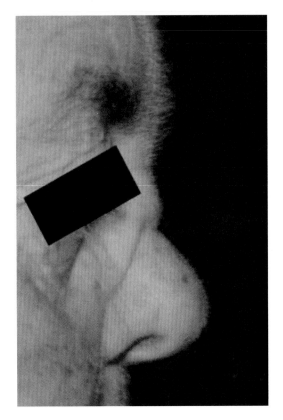

FIGURE 18.2 Nasal collapse in a patient with RP

18.5.3   Pulmonary

Dyspnoea with stridor is suggestive of tracheal involvement. Respiratory involvement is the most serious complication of RP and occurs in up to 50 % of patients. Tenderness may be present over the trachea and thyroid cartilage. Recurrent laryngeal and tracheal inflammation leads to hoarseness, dry cough, dyspnoea, wheeze, and stridor. Involvement of the larynx and epiglottis may lead to upper airway collapse, which can require emergency tracheostomy.

18.5.4   Ophthalmic

Painful red eyes with blurred vision suggest the development of scleritis or episcleritis. There may be recurrent episodes of episcleritis or scleritis, conjunctivitis, keratitis and uveitis. Slit lamp examination is required to formally assess the extent of ocular inflammation.

18.5.5   Musculoskeletal

Joint pain is a common feature. This can involve both large and small joints and the axial skeleton.

18.5.6   Cutaneous

Skin involvement is common with purpura, papules, aphthosis, and pustules.

18.5.7   Cardiovascular

Cardiovascular involvement is uncommon. The most common involvement is complete heart block, aortic valve rupture, and acute aortic regurgitation.

18.6   Laboratory Features

The diagnosis is usually made on the characteristic clinical features. Investigation is directed at establishing the diagnosis and assessing the extent and severity of organ involvement. There is evidence of inflammation with the elevation of ESR and CRP.

18.6.1   Immunology

ANCA, ANA, RF, anticardiolipin and anti-GBM antibodies are usually negative. Complement levels are normal. Cryoglobulins are not detected negative.

18.6.2   Imaging

Airway collapse can be visualized using fast sequence CT scanning, which permits dynamic assessment. Eighteen FDG-PET-CT may be used to establish extent of disease.

18.6.3   Pathology

Biopsy of the ear shows a perichondritis with the presence of mononuclear cells and occasional polymorphonuclear leucocytes at the fibrochondral junction. A skin biopsy may show a leucocytoclastic or lymphocytic vasculitis.

18.7   Diagnosis

The diagnosis is based on the typical clinical features. The differential diagnosis is from other types of chondritis and perichondritis. Infection may lead to perichondritis. Granulomatosis with polyangiitis (Wegener's) and lethal midline granuloma may lead to nasal destruction. The Mouth And Genital ulcers with Inflamed Cartilage (MAGIC) syndrome is an overlap between RP and Behçet's disease.

18.8   Assessment Disease Activity

There are no formal assessment tools for disease activity. ESR and CRP provide a guide to activity, but are non are specific. Regular respiratory function testing may provide evidence of laryngeal involvement.

18.9   Treatment

There are no randomized controlled trials in RP. Only NSAIDs only are adequate for patients with mild chondritis. Laryngotracheal involvement requires glucocorticoids at high doses (prednisolone 0.5–1.0 mg/kg) [2, 3]. Long-term maintenance therapy may be required to control inflammation. Immunosuppression with methotrexate, azathioprine, leflunomide and ciclosporin has been reported to be effective in controlling chronic inflammation and is used when control of disease can not be maintained with oral glucocorticoids. The role of TNF-alpha blockade, anti-IL-6 therapy, abatercept and B cell depletion is still to be determined, but encouraging reports are available [4, 5].

Acute airway obstruction refractory to medical treatment may require tracheostomy. Patients with tracheal collapse may be managed with stents.

18.10   Prognosis

The course is usually relapsing and remitting. The mortality is low at 6 % at 8 years. Most patients develop some disability with hearing or visual impairment, speech impediment. There is a risk of myelodysplasia.

Key Points
- Rare condition characterized by inflammation and destruction of cartilage.
- Inflammation typically involves the nasal and auricular cartilage.
- Upper airway inflammation may lead to obstruction requiring urgent tracheostomy.

References

1. Michet C, McKeena CH, Luthra HS, O'Fallon WM. Relapsing polychondritis. Survival and predictive role of early disease manifestations. Ann Intern Med. 1986;104:74–8.
2. Staats BA, Utz JP, Michet CJ. Relapsing polychondritis. Semin Respir Crit Care Med. 2002;23:145–54.

3. Gergely P, Poor G. Relapsing polychondritis. Best Pract Res Clin Rheumatol. 2004;18:723–38.
4. Leroux G, Costedoat-Chalulmeau N, Brihaye N, et al. Treatment of relapsing polychondritis with rituximab – a retrospective study of nine patients. Arthritis Rheum. 2009;61:577–82.
5. Loricera J, Blanco R, Castaneda S, et al. Tocilizumab in refractory aortitis: a study on 16 cases and a literature review. Clin Exp Rheumatol. 2014;32:S79–89.

Chapter 19
Cogan's Syndrome

19.1 Introduction

Cogan's syndrome (CS) is a rare inflammatory disease of unknown etiology, characterized by the involvement of the eye and inner ear.

19.2 Definition and Classification

There are no validated diagnostic criteria or classification criteria.

19.3 Epidemiology

The incidence and prevalence of CS are unknown, but it occurs mainly in young adults with a peak incidence in those aged 20–30 years. There is no gender predominance.

19.4 Etiology

The etiology is unknown, but like many autoimmune conditions, is generally believed to result from an environmental trigger interacting with a genetically predisposed host. Infection

R.A. Watts et al., *Vasculitis in Clinical Practice*,
DOI 10.1007/978-3-319-14871-7_19,
© Springer International Publishing AG, Cham 2015

has long been suspected as a trigger, but not proven. The eye and the ear are both capable of mounting a vigorous response to infection, trauma, or toxins. In an experimental model of autoimmune keratitis in rats, transfer of corneal specific T cells produces a severe keratitis. Similarly, transfer of activated T cells can induce vestibular inflammation in animal models.

19.5   Clinical Features

The combination of ocular and vestibular symptoms in a young adult should raise a suspicion of CS [1–3].

19.5.1   Systemic

The initial symptoms may be nonspecific with fever, weight loss and fatigue.

19.5.2   Ocular

The predominant complaints are of ocular pain, redness and photophobia. Blurring of vision, tearing, diplopia, a sensation of foreign body or visual field defects occur frequently. Slit lamp examination is necessary to observe interstitial keratitis, which occurs in 70 % of patients. The earliest findings are faint corneal infiltrates which are 0.5–1 mm in diameter. Other frequent manifestations are conjunctivitis (35 %), iridocyclitis (30 %) and episcleritis/scleritis (30 %). Less common features include posterior uveitis, and papillitis.

19.5.3   Vestibular and Auditory

The typical features are sudden onset of vertigo, nausea, vomiting, tinnitus and hearing loss. Attacks are similar to Meniere's disease. Hearing loss occurs in 95 %, ataxia (45 %), nystagmus (30 %), and oscillopsia (15 %).

19.5.4   Vascular

Symptoms of vasculitis depend on the territory and size of vessel involved. Any size of vessel may be involved. Large vessel vasculitis akin to Takayasu arteritis is most common. An aortitis occurs in 10 % with severe aortic regurgitation. Pericarditis and arrhythmias are less common.

19.5.5   Neurological

Neurological involvement is uncommon in CS, but its features include meningitis, encephalitis, psychosis, and seizures.

19.6   Laboratory Features

The diagnosis is usually made on the characteristic clinical features. Investigation is directed at establishing the diagnosis and assessing the extent and severity of organ involvement. There is evidence of inflammation with the elevation of ESR and CRP.

19.6.1   Immunology

ANCA, ANA, RF, anticardiolipin, and anti-GBM antibodies are usually negative. Complement levels are normal. Cryoglobulins are not detected.

19.6.2   Pathology

Corneal biopsies may show a plasma cell infiltrate and lymphocytes in the deeper layers of the cornea with scarring and neovascularization. The histology of vessels is similar to that seen in GCA, with an inflammatory infiltrate, intimal proliferation, disruption of the internal elastic lamina, and multinucleate giant cells.

19.7   Diagnosis

CS should be considered in any patient presenting with ocular inflammation and evidence of audiovestibular dysfunction. The differential diagnosis is from other types of vasculitis, which may cause scleritis or uveitis (granulomatosis with polyangiitis (Wegener's), polyarteritis nodosa, Behçet's disease).

19.8   Assessment of Disease Activity

Slit lamp examination is necessary to examine the anterior chamber and cornea. Fluoroscein angiography is useful to assess retinal vasculitis or retinochoroiditis.

Audiometry is necessary to assess the severity of hearing loss. Ninety-five percent of patients have hearing loss, with relative sparing of the middle range. Brainstem evoked responses are abnormal in patients with cochlear damage. Caloric responses are abnormal with vestibular injury.

19.9   Treatment

There are no controlled trials of therapy in CS. Glucocorticoids are the mainstay of treatment for acute flares and recurrences of ocular and auditory inflammation. Keratitis and anterior uveitis usually respond to topical glucocorticoids. Posterior scleritis and retinitis require oral glucocorticoids. Audiovestibular disease requires high dose oral glucocorticoids (prednisone 1–2 mg/kg/day). Resistant disease requires immunosuppression with methotrexate; ciclosporin, azathioprine, tacrolimus and cyclophosphamide have all been tried. The role of TNF blockade and B cell depletion remains to be determined.

19.10   Prognosis

There is an initial flare, which may last several weeks to months, followed by a chronic slowly progressive phase. Ocular outcomes are good. Blindness occurs in <5 % of eyes. Deafness is a frequent and debilitating outcome occurring in up to 54 % of patients. Corticosteroids may improve the outcome. Vestibular manifestations improve for most patients. Large vessel vasculitis with aortic incompetence can be associated with a poor prognosis.

> **Key Points**
> - Rare condition characterized by ocular and auditory inflammation
> - Deafness is the most common long term sequelae.

References

1. Grasland A, Pouchout J, Hachulla E, Bletry O, Papo T, Vinceneux P. Study Group for Cogan's Syndrome. Typical and atypical Cogan's syndrome: 32 cases and review of the literature. Rheumatology. 2004;43:1007–15.
2. Mazlumzadeh M, Matteson EL. Cogan's syndrome: an audiovestibular, ocular, and systemic autoimmune disease. Rheum Dis Clin North Am. 2007;33:855–74.
3. Greco A, Gallo A, Fusconi M, et al. Cogan's syndrome an autoimmune inner ear disease. Autoimmun Rev. 2013;12:396–400.

Chapter 20
IgG4 Related Disease

20.1 Introduction

Peripheral levels of IgG4 were seen to be elevated in patients with cystic fibrosis and atopic dermatitis in the 1970s [1, 2]. Shakib et al. hypothesized that this phenomenon implicated the role of IgG4 in immediate type hypersensitivity disorders. Raised IgG4 levels in the context of a vasculitis syndrome were demonstrated in the 1980s [3, 4]. The term 'IgG4 related autoimmune disease' was first proposed by Kamisawa et al. when referring to autoimmune pancreatitis and its related diseases [5]. Retroperitoneal fibrosis in 2002 [6], and subsequently aortitis in 2008 [7] have been recognised to be part of the spectrum of this multi-organ disease.

20.2 Definition and Classification

As a relatively newly described condition, there is no recognised definition or classification criteria. It is accepted that this condition is a result of lymphoplasmacytic infiltration of tissues with IgG4 positive plasma cells resulting in 'storiform' fibrosis and obliterative phlebitis.

R.A. Watts et al., *Vasculitis in Clinical Practice*,
DOI 10.1007/978-3-319-14871-7_20,
© Springer International Publishing AG, Cham 2015

20.3   Epidemiology

There are no reliable figures for the incidence of this condition due to inconsistency of nomenclature. The majority of literature around this condition has emerged from Japan, and therefore it is thought to be commoner in the Japanese. Various features of IgG4 related disease may have different gender predisposition. Ophthalmopathy appears to have equal gender distribution [8], but non-head and neck manifestations appear to be predominantly in men in the sixth and seventh decades of life [9].

20.4   Aetiology

The aetiology is unknown. There is evidence of immune complex deposition in cases with autoimmune pancreatitis [10]. No autoantigenic target has been isolated. Allergy and hypersensitivity may have a role to play. IgG4 has long been thought to play a role in allergic tolerance [11]. Several HLA and non-HLA genes have been associated with IgG4 related disease [12].

20.5   Clinical Features

IgG4 related disease has been recognised in a large number of sites.

20.5.1   Ocular Disease

Unilateral or bilateral proptosis due to retro-orbital pseudo-tumour can occur. Lacrimal gland inflammation will cause periorbital swelling and dry eyes.

20.5.2   Salivary Gland Involvement

Unilateral or bilateral salivary gland enlargement with sicca syndrome can be a feature. A proportion of patients who fulfil the classification criteria for Sjogren's syndrome have been shown to have elevated IgG4 levels [13].

20.5.3 Thyroid Involvement

This can present either as Reidel's thyroiditis or Hashimoto's thyroiditis.

20.5.4 Pulmonary Involvement

Cases may present with a chronic cough, haemoptysis, dyspnoea or pleuritic chest pain. Fibrotic lung or pleural disease may occur. The radiological appearances may be discrete nodular or diffuse interstitial. Honeycombing and ground-glass changes can be seen.

20.5.5 Aortic and Periaortic Involvement

IgG4 related disease can result in inflammatory aneurysms of the thoracic and abdominal aorta [7, 14].

20.5.6 Pancreatico-Biliary Involvement

Autoimmune pancreatitis can present with a pancreatic mass or painless jaundice. It may present as diabetes mellitus. Sclerosing cholangitis due to IgG4 related disease may be difficult to differentiate from primary sclerosing cholangitis or cholangiocarcinoma. The cholangiopathy almost never occurs before pancreatic involvement.

20.5.7 Urological Involvement

Tubulointerstitial nephritis may present with renal function or urinary abnormalities. Obstructive uropathy due to retroperitoneal fibrosis may occur. Prostatitis has been described.

20.6   Laboratory Features

20.6.1   Haematology Tests

The full blood count is consistent with acute phase response. The erythrocyte sedimentation rate is usually significantly elevated. Circulating levels of plasmablasts are elevated. This may serve as a biomarker of disease activity.

20.6.2   Serum Biochemistry

Obstructive liver function may be suggestive of pancreatico-biliary involvement. Renal function may be impaired due to tubulo-interstitial nephritis or obstructive uropathy.

20.6.3   Immunology

A number of patients may have low-tire presence of antinuclear antibodies and rheumatoid factor [15]. The serum IgG4 levels are elevated in 85 % of cases [9].

20.6.4   Urine Analysis

Asymptomatic proteinuria may be a sign of tubulointerstitial nephritis.

20.6.5   Imaging

Computed tomography of various organs will delineate the nature of the disease – discrete nodular or diffuse fibrotic. However, positron emission tomography is 'hot' in the affected organs.

20.6.6   Tissue Biopsy

The presence of a dense lymphoplasmacytic infiltrate with storiform (cart-wheel) fibrosis and obliterative phlebitis is classic. Large numbers of plasma cells stain positive for IgG4. Tissue IgG4 positive plasma cells are more specific than serum IgG4 elevation.

20.7   Diagnosis

The spectrum of IgG4 related disease has been continuously widening over the past few years. This must be suspected in a wide variety of patients – from the generally unwell with acute phase response to the obviously jaundiced with evidence of pancreatico-biliary involvement. This should be in the differential diagnosis of patients with salivary gland and/or lacrimal gland involvement, pancreatitis, aortitis and proptosis.

20.7.1   Assessment of Disease Activity

Serum IgG4 levels and inflammatory markers may serve as general markers of disease activity. In the absence of any validated specific biomarker, careful clinical evaluation will be the basis of assessing disease activity.

20.8   Treatment

There is very little evidence for formulating a strategy. Glucocorticoid therapy usually results in rapid normalisation of inflammatory markers. The typical dose of prednisolone is 1 mg/kg/day (max 60 mg), reduced to 15 mg/day by 3 months. All titration should be accompanied by careful clinical evaluation. The ultimate goal should be withdrawal of glucocorticoid therapy. There is an increasing trend to use Rituximab in patients who become glucocorticoid dependent or relapse on withdrawal of glucocorticoid therapy. The plasma cell population from lymph nodes of patients with IgG4 related disease has been shown to express CD20 [16]. In open labelled use, Rituximab 1 g×2 pulses, 2 weeks apart was associated with clinical improvement and lowered serum IgG4 levels [17]. There is anecdotal evidence for the benefit of using methotrexate, azathioprine, mycophenolate mofetil and cyclophosphamide.

20.9   Prognosis

The prognosis of this condition has not been defined adequately. It would be reasonable to assume that this is related to the extent of organ involvement. For example, patients with pure salivary gland involvement are likely to do better than those with autoimmune pancreatitis or inflammatory aortic aneurysms. IgG4 related disease does not appear to be related to a higher risk of cancer [18].

Key Points
- IgG4 related disease is a new fibro-inflammatory disease with a myriad of organ involvement, all of which were thought to previously be disparate conditions.
- It is associated with a rise in tissue and circulating IgG4 levels, lymphoplasmacytic tissue infiltrate, storiform (cartwheel) fibrosis producing either discrete lesions or diffuse fibrosis.
- The condition is responsive to glucocorticoid therapy and rituximab may be the ideal drug to treat this condition long-term.

References

1. Shakib F, Stanworth DR, Smalley CA, Brown GA. Elevated serum IgG4 levels in cystic fibrosis patients. Clin Allergy. 1976;6(3):237–40.

2. Shakib F, McLaughlan P, Stanworth DR, Smith E, Fairburn E. Elevated serum IgE and IgG4 in patients with atopic dermatitis. Br J Dermatol. 1977;97(1):59–63.

3. van Nieuwkoop JA, Brand A, Radl J, Skvaril F. Increased levels of IgG4 subclass in 5 patients with acquired respiratory disease. Int Arch Allergy Appl Immunol. 1982;67(1):61–5.

4. Oxelius VA. Immunoglobulin G, (IgG) subclasses and human disease. Am J Med. 1984;76(3A):7–18.

5. Kamisawa T, Funata N, Hayashi Y, Eishi Y, Koike M, Tsuruta K, et al. A new clinicopathological entity of IgG4-related autoimmune disease. J Gastroenterol. 2003;38(10):982–4.

6. Hamano H, Kawa S, Ochi Y, Unno H, Shiba N, Wajiki M, et al. Hydronephrosis associated with retroperitoneal fibrosis and sclerosing pancreatitis. Lancet. 2002;359(9315):1403–4.

7. Kasashima S, Zen Y, Kawashima A, Konishi K, Sasaki H, Endo M, et al. Inflammatory abdominal aortic aneurysm: close relationship to IgG4-related periaortitis. Am J Surg Pathol. 2008;32(2):197–204.

8. Japanese study group of IgG4-related ophthalmic disease. Jpn J Ophthalmol. 2013;57(6):573–9.

9. Zen Y, Nakanuma Y. IgG4-related disease: a cross-sectional study of 114 cases. Am J Surg Pathol. 2010;34(12):1812–9.

10. Deshpande V, Chicano S, Finkelberg D, Selig MK, Mino-Kenudson M, Brugge WR, et al. Autoimmune pancreatitis: a systemic immune complex mediated disease. Am J Surg Pathol. 2006;30(12):1537–45.

11. Gwynn CM, Smith JM, Leon GL, Stanworth DR. Role of IgG4 subclass in childhood allergy. Lancet. 1978;1(8070):910–1.

12. Zen Y, Nakanuma Y. Pathogenesis of IgG4-related disease. Curr Opin Rheumatol. 2011;23(1):114–8.

13. Mavragani CP, Fragoulis GE, Rontogianni D, Kanariou M, Moutsopoulos HM. Elevated IgG4 serum levels among primary Sjogren's syndrome patients: do they unmask underlying IgG4-related disease? Arthritis Care Res (Hoboken). 2014;66(5):773–7.

14. Agaimy A, Weyand M, Strecker T. Inflammatory thoracic aortic aneurysm (lymphoplasmacytic thoracic aortitis): a 13-year-experience at a German Heart Center with emphasis on possible role of IgG4. Int J Clin Exp Pathol. 2013;6(9):1713–22.

15. Song TJ, Kim MH, Moon SH, Eum JB, Park do H, Lee SS, et al. The combined measurement of total serum IgG and IgG4 may increase diagnostic sensitivity for autoimmune pancreatitis without sacrificing specificity, compared with IgG4 alone. Am J Gastroenterol. 2010;105(7):1655–60.

16. Grimm KE, Bakke A, O'Malley DP. Abnormal expression of CD20 on IgG4 plasma cells associated with IgG4-related lymphadenopathy. Arch Pathol Lab Med. 2013;137(9):1282–5.

17. Khosroshahi A, Bloch DB, Deshpande V, Stone JH. Rituximab therapy leads to rapid decline of serum IgG4 levels and prompt clinical improvement in IgG4-related systemic disease. Arthritis Rheum. 2010;62(6):1755–62.

18. Hirano K, Tada M, Sasahira N, Isayama H, Mizuno S, Takagi K, et al. Incidence of malignancies in patients with IgG4-related disease. Intern Med. 2014;53(3):171–6.

Index

R.A. Watts et al., *Vasculitis in Clinical Practice*,
DOI 10.1007/978-3-319-14871-7,
© Springer International Publishing AG, Cham 2015